Slimmer and Trimmer

Slimmer and Trimmer

Daily Tips for Permanent Weight Loss

Arpi A. Simonian, MS, ScM

VANTAGE PRESS
New York

The guidelines promoted in this program are similar to the recommendations of the Dietary Guidelines for Americans by the United States Department of Agriculture, The Surgeon General's Report on Nutrition and Health by the United States Department of Health and Human Services, and the American Heart Association.

In addition to promoting permanent weight loss, these guidelines help in the prevention and treatment of hypertension, heart disease, and other health problems that are related to weight and diet.

Readers are advised to consult their own personal physicians before starting this or any other weight-control program, and before making any major changes in their diet or activity level, especially if they suffer from chest pain, joint pain, shortness of breath, or if they have a medical problem, such as diabetes, high blood pressure, or heart disease.

The author wishes to thank Oldways Preservation & Exchange Trust for permission to reprint the illustration on page 282. Their website is http://oldwayspt.org.

FIRST EDITION

Published by Vantage Press, Inc.
516 West 34th Street, New York, New York 10001

Manufactured in the United States of America
ISBN: 0-533-14511-2

Library of Congress Catalog Card No.: 2002096893

0 9 8 7 6 5 4 3 2 1

Respectfully dedicated to you, dear reader, for taking the initiative to lead a healthier and happier life.

Topics Covered

Fats and Oils
Reducing Fat Intake

Protein
The Healthier Protein Sources

Carbohydrates
The Undesirable Simple Carbohydrates
The Good Complex Carbohydrates

Physical Activity
Walking

Calories

Goal Setting

Behavior Modification
Good Eating Habits
Buying, Preparing, Serving, Storing Food
Eating Out, Vacations, Celebrations

Self-reliance
Keeping Records

Weight Maintenance

Children
Establishing Good Eating Habits Early On

Author's Note

Your Daily Companion

—Put into practice one new tip a day.
—Adopt a new nutrition guideline.
—Make small but permanent changes in your eating habits.
—Gradually modify the foods you eat.
—Increase your physical activity and become the fit person you can be.
—Take charge and improve your image.

Acknowledgments

My deepest gratitude to all the eminent physiologists, biochemists, nutritionists, psychologists, psychiatrists, physicians, cardiologists, and physical trainers who carried out the scientific research and clinical studies and produced the wealth of information about weight control and healthy living that we promote and practice in this program.

Introduction: Weight Control for a Lifetime

Slimmer and Trimmer introduces one new tip per day for permanent weight loss. It incorporates all four contributing factors in weight control, namely nutrition education, behavior modification, physical activity, and self-reliance. It synthesizes the available scientific knowledge and translates it into simple and practical steps that are easy to incorporate into everyday life. It is a plan to promote fundamental, long-term, and enjoyable changes in your lifestyle.

Minor daily changes will guide you to strengthen your motivation, enjoy new healthy eating habits, permanently modify your food preferences, incorporate physical activity into your routine, and attain the weight loss and fitness you desire. The focus is on gradually shaping and evolving a new trim, active, and happy self.

The innovative approach of offering one practical idea a day, as well as tips for raising healthy children, sets this apart from other books in the diet field. This motivating program covers an entire year. You can start at any time during the year.

Day 1

Fat

The amount of fat that Americans consume is enormous, by historic standards, when compared to human dietary traditions of the past.

The average American diet contains more than twice, and in some cases three times, the fat we need for our daily energy requirements. The excess fat is stored in our body around muscles, under the skin, in and around vital organs and in the arteries, and it can cause hypertension, cardiovascular diseases, and other health hazards.

Reducing fat intake is crucial for weight reduction and healthier living. Decrease the amount of fat that you eat in whatever form or shape.

Day 2

Fat

Fats and oils are found in foods from both animal and plant sources. Fats and oils are used in obvious forms such as butter, margarine, shortening, cooking oil and salad oil, which are added during food preparation.

Fats and oils are also found in less obvious forms inherent in meat, nuts, seeds and dairy products such as whole milk, ice cream, and cheese.

Gradually reduce and eventually eliminate the fats and oils used at the table during meals. Enjoy the delicious taste of the dinner roll and the distinct flavors of your vegetables without adding butter.

Do not use or serve butter at the table.

Day 3

Fat

Fats from animal sources, such as butter, meat cuts, lard, suet, and chicken are generally solid at room temperature and as a result are easier to detect and easier to eliminate from the diet.

Trim all visible fat from raw meat and poultry before preparing food.

Remove all visible fat and skin from cooked meat or poultry before eating.

Day 4

Behavior

Are popcorn, soda, and candy bars an indispensable part of going to the movie theater? Do you go to the movies immediately after dinner, and take along that box of popcorn oozing with butter, just because that's what you have always done?

Think about it!

Instead of remaining the slave of your old habits, eliminate them by choice. Avoid eating at the movies. You are busy watching anyway.

People do not snack at the opera or during the performance of the symphony orchestra, and they all survive elegantly.

Day 5

Protein

Protein is an essential nutrient. It helps build muscles and body tissues, and is vital especially for growing children and adolescents. A healthy and balanced diet should include protein for good nutrition, but only in moderation.

The average American diet contains twice, sometimes three times, the protein necessary for good nutrition.

Eat smaller portions of meat and poultry.

Day 6

Protein

More than two-thirds of the protein in the average American diet originates from animal flesh, especially beef. We generally tend to equate the word "protein" with "beef."

Remember that poultry, fish, and shellfish are equally good sources of protein and have the additional advantage of lower fat content.

When possible, choose a small portion of turkey, chicken, or fish instead of beef.

Day 7

Choosing the Right Meat

6 ounces of	Calories	Fat grams
Turkey breast	270	5
Chicken breast, no skin	275	7
Dark-meat chicken, no skin	390	15
Veal	395	20
Darkmeat chicken, with skin	430	25
Sirloin steak, broiled	460	30
Ground beef, broiled	460	30
Pork loin, braised	530	35

Make the wiser choices. Select the ones that contain less fat and fewer calories.

Day 8

The Power Within

You have within you the power to lose weight and keep it off forever.

Yes, you can do it. You can lose weight naturally and stay trim for good.

You have already learned the hard way that there are no effective gimmicks, miracle fad diets, or safe magic pills. Admit the sobering fact that **in order to lose weight and keep it off for good, small, gradual but permanent changes must be made in your entire lifestyle.**

You can transform your life and realize your dream.

Day 9

Carbohydrates

Carbohydrates are the principal sources of energy for the body. They contain about four calories per gram, the same as proteins and about half as much as fats. Sources of carbohydrate are plentiful in nature and cost less than sources of protein or fat.

Fad diets have done a disservice by claiming carbohydrates as foods to be avoided completely, because they do not make the crucial distinction between the undesirable carbohydrates, known as **"Simple Carbohydrates"** and the good carbohydrates, **"Complex Carbohydrates."**

Day 10

Simple Carbohydrates

These are the highly refined and processed sugars, honey, molasses and syrups, often eaten in concentrated form as candy, sweets, candy bars, chocolate, cakes, and other desserts. These are poor in nutrients and high in calories.

It is this category that has given carbohydrates a bad name. **Avoid using these simple carbohydrates or reduce their intake to the minimum.**

Day 11

Complex Carbohydrates

These are found in fruits and vegetables and in starchy foods—such as potatoes, cereals, breads, pastas, and beans.

Contrary to popular belief, foods high in complex carbohydrates are among the best foods you can eat. They are most valuable when minimally processed or refined, especially when closest to their natural form, such as fresh fruit, raw vegetables, whole grain cereals, brown rice (only husk removed), un-milled grains (vitamins, minerals, and fiber still intact) and whole grain breads.

Replace part of the meat in your diet with these complex carbohydrates whenever possible.

Day 12

Portion Control

The average American eats too much.

The amount of food served at home, at receptions, and in restaurants is enormous—way beyond the body's requirement for nutrition and energy.

In addition to these generous servings, the unnecessary snacking between meals has become routine.

Modify your habit of automatic overeating, and gradually reduce the excessive amount of your servings.

Day 13

Restaurant Portions

Restaurants have increased the size of their servings in their effort to lure and satisfy patrons. Some even present food to individuals in overflowing oval serving platters. As a result people simply eat too much.

The all-you-can-eat buffet settings are even more hazardous to your weight, your waist, and your health. These offerings encourage mindless overindulgence, thus contributing to undesirable weight gain.

Do not stuff yourself with more than your body needs for nutrition and energy. Eat small portions.

Day 14

Calories

The balance between food intake and energy expenditure determines weight changes.

Similar to your savings account, in which if you

—deposit more than you withdraw, your balance increases, or if you
—withdraw and spend more than you deposit, your savings dwindle.

In your body, if your

—food energy intake is more than your total energy expenditure, your fat deposits increase, or if you
—burn up more than you eat, you lose weight.

Day 15

Calories

If your weight has been imperceptibly but ever so consistently creeping up year after year, you are definitely eating more than your body needs for healthy living and normal activity. You are taking in excess calories.

To maintain your weight, limit your calorie intake to the level of the total calories burned. To lose weight**, decrease total calorie intake further, or compensate by increasing physical activity.**

Eat smaller portions than in the past.

Day 16

Energy

The living body requires a continuous supply of energy to perform the specific functions of all the internal organs, to maintain the physiologic and biochemical balances, to develop new tissue in growing children and adolescents, and to carry on body movement and physical activities of all kinds.

Increase your exercise. The additional physical activity burns up extra calories, thus using up more of your body's fat deposits to provide the energy necessary.

Lace up your sneakers and get out there!

Day 17

Physical Activity

Our miraculous and wonderful body and physiology evolved over the millenniums with physical activity as an integral, routine and inseparable part of life. **Incorporate some form of physical activity in your life, as part of your daily routine, for better weight control and overall healthy living. Discover the joy of feeling fit!**

Day 18

Physical Activity Is Vital

You put on weight not only because you overeat, but also because you lead a sedentary life. Both food intake and physical activity influence your weight.

Decreasing food consumption and limiting calorie intake help you lose the fat.

Similarly, increased physical activity helps you burn the fat and decrease the fat deposits. Decreasing food intake and increasing activity complement each other to lose the extra fat.

Day 19

Physical Activity

If you are leading a completely sedentary life, then you will agree it is time to give another lifestyle a fair chance. **Your body deserves better care. Think of exercise as a special gift to yourself.**

Choose an activity that you will enjoy. Physical activity should be pleasant, accessible, available, and inexpensive. You have a wide variety of aerobic exercises and many sports to choose from: swimming, tennis, dance, bicycling, and many, many more.

Begin your journey to fitness and fun.

Day 20

Walking

If the idea of physical activity seems too traumatic, **start by walking. Yes, WALKING.**

Walking is a natural and invigorating activity for our body, as normal as eating and sleeping. **In addition to burning up calories, walking assists the heart in blood circulation** through the constant movements of the legs. When the large leg muscles contract rhythmically, they help pump the blood back to the heart.

Be good to yourself—go for a walk.

Day 21

Think Positive

Believe in yourself. Believe that you can do it. Trust that you have within you the power to reshape your body and your life. When you have a "can do" attitude, nothing can stop you.

Congratulate yourself for having demonstrated such determination and discipline in making this serious commitment.

Start visualizing how trim you will look and how good you will be feeling.

You can be rightfully proud of yourself for taking up this mature challenge.

Day 22

Weight Control

Effective weight control is achieved by a combination of:

—Dietary modifications
—Eating behavior improvement
—Regular physical activity
—Self management

Follow the daily tips presented and you will be making fundamental improvements in all these parameters that are an integral part of weight control.

Day 23

Behavior

The habit of watching television during meals creates the mental association of the two activities. As a result, watching television conditions you to reach for a snack regardless of the fact that you might not be hungry at all.

Are you associating television viewing with eating? Have you programmed yourself to reach for a snack when you settle down in front of the television set, in spite of the fact that you just had dinner?

Eating should be an independent activity.
Do not watch television while eating.
Do not eat while watching television.

Day 24

Liquid Fillers

Make it a habit to begin each meal by drinking a "liquid filler": a glass of water, sparkling water, diet beverage, iced tea, herb tea, or other low-calorie liquids. Fresh lemon or lime squeezed in a glass of cold water makes an ideal healthy drink.

Take sips of water between bites. This has the dual advantage of slowing down eating and simultaneously adding volume to the stomach, promoting the feeling of "fullness."

Day 25

EAT SLOWLY

Hunger is controlled by the brain and is caused by a drop in the level of blood sugars. Food intake raises the concentration of blood sugars. The higher amount of sugar in the blood alerts the brain and thus alleviates hunger.

But there is a twenty-minute time lag between the satiation in the stomach and the awareness of relief of hunger in the brain. So if you gobble down your food, you will eat more than necessary to "feel full."

Slow down and linger over a leisurely meal.

Day 26

Travel

Have you ever realized how on long trips you stock the car with food, snacks, and drinks and end up eating continuously "to pass the time" as if eating were a form of entertainment?

To beat boredom or break the monotony of the long drive, keep up a lively conversation with your companions in the car. If driving alone, take along some books-on-tape from the public library, or some self-help tapes and make it an enjoyable learning experience.

Keep all food and snacks in the trunk, make planned mealtime stops, and enjoy.

Day 27

Buying Food

Each one of us has had the much too common experience of walking into the grocery store with the intention of buying just two items and walking out with two overflowing grocery bags.

Always go marketing prepared with a written grocery list. This will discourage impulsive buying of the fattening foods that you are trying to avoid.

Day 28

Serving Food

No casserole or serving platter on the table.

A serving platter of food on the table in full view and within easy reach of diners is an invitation for overeating.

Keep casseroles, pots, and serving platters warm in the kitchen, away from the table. This practice will help avoid reaching out for additional helpings just because the food is at your fingertips and accessible.

Day 29

Eating Out

Avoid "all you can eat" buffet settings if you cannot resist the temptation of the abundant display of food settings or if you have difficulty limiting your portions. Stay away from buffet brunches if you succumb to the feeling that you must get your money's worth by eating until you are "totally stuffed."

Choose the restaurant wisely. Call ahead to inquire about the menu and patronize the restaurants that offer "light" or "healthy" items.

Day 30

Rewards

Make sure you look your best at all times. Change your grooming to reflect your confident new self and active lifestyle.

Indulge in a new hairstyle. Be bold. Experiment with the fashionable younger look that you have been contemplating for some time. Choose a style that will complement and emphasize your good looks.

You have earned the right to draw attention to yourself, your attractive physical features, and happy disposition.

Day 31

Weighing Yourself

To keep track of your progress, weigh yourself once a week, first thing in the morning. For your convenience, a chart is provided at the end of this book.

If you feel that weighing yourself each morning works as a daily reminder to reinforce your motivation, your commitment and your resolve, then by all means, go ahead and weigh yourself each morning. Do what works best for you. Remember, however, that weight can fluctuate as much as three pounds due to water retention.

Day 32

Set a Goal for Yourself

Determine how much you want to weigh, what size clothing you would like to wear, and what activities you will take up. Your goal should be based on your own perception of yourself, not on some suggested weight tables or averages. **The most important consideration is that you feel comfortable with yourself, that you feel good about the way you look, and that the image you project is compatible with the happy and active person you are.**

Write down your goal and refer to it regularly.

Day 33

Current Diet

The trouble with the current American diet is that there is:

—Too much total fat
—Too much animal flesh
—Too much processed food
—Too much sugar and salt
—Too little fruit and vegetables
—Too little cereal and legumes
—Too little fiber

Make a strong commitment to correct these unhealthy trends. You owe it to yourself!

Day 34

A Healthy Balance

The nutrients that the body needs in order to fulfill the requirements for healthy living are provided by the different components of the foods we eat: fats, proteins, carbohydrates, vitamins, minerals, and water.

The average American diet runs to about 40-50 percent of total calories in fat, 15-20 percent in protein and 35-45 percent in carbohydrates. In some cases, fat constitutes almost half of the total calorie intake.

We should strive towards 15-25 percent fat, 10-25 percent protein, and 55-65 percent complex carbohydrates for adults.

Day 35

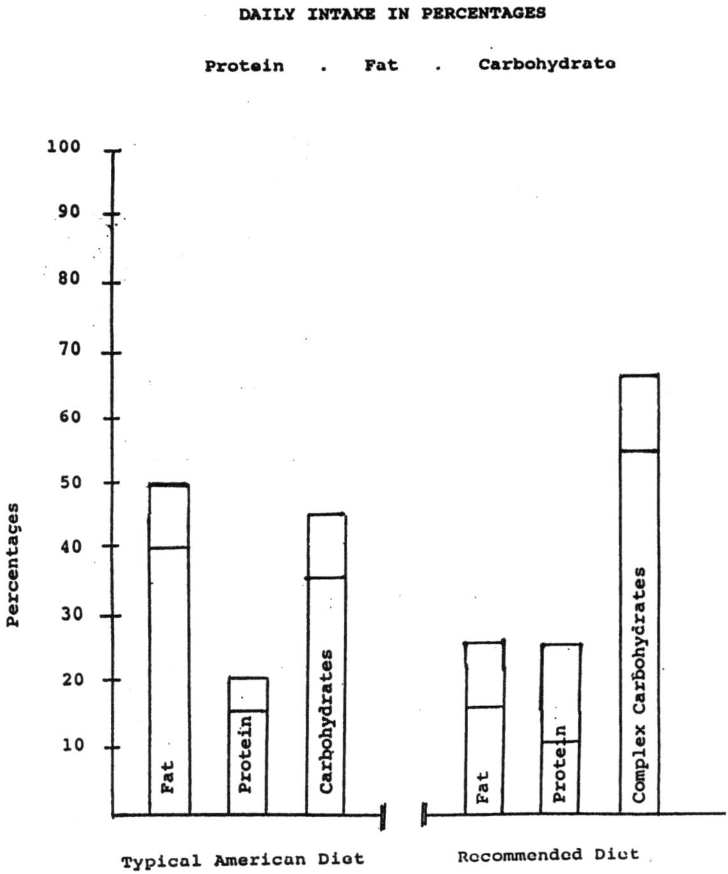
DAILY INTAKE IN PERCENTAGES
Protein . Fat . Carbohydrate
100
90
80
70
60
50
40
30
20
10
Percentages
Fat
Protein
Carbohydrates
Fat
Protein
Complex Carbohydrates
Typical American Diet
Recommended Diet

Day 36

Fat

Most foods naturally contain some fat. Even when you eliminate the use of butter and oil in cooking, you will still be taking in 10 to 15 percent of your total calories from fat. Hence you must reduce the addition of fats and oils to the bare minimum.

When preparing food, **make it a habit to decrease the amount of fat used. Cut the amount of butter, margarine, or oil indicated in your recipe by half. As your taste buds adjust, decrease fats to a third, and eventually to a quarter.** You will be delighted to realize that you will enjoy your food more than ever before.

Embrace the wiser and healthier alternative.

Day 37

Fat

There are three major categories of fat, based on their chemical structure:

1. Saturated fat comes mainly from animal sources. The fat found in meat and dairy products contains relatively high ratios of saturated fat. Some plant oils, such as coconut oil and palm oil, contain high amounts of saturated fat too.

2. Monounsaturated fat comes from plant sources such as avocadoes and olive oil.

3. Polyunsaturated fat is found mostly in vegetable oils and fish oils.

Saturated fat is the category to be used sparingly.

Day 38

Compare

	Approximate Fat Grams per Cup	Approximate Calories per Cup
Creamed Cottage Cheese	4	240
Low-fat Cottage Cheese	2	180
Low-fat Cottage Cheese	1	160
Ice Cream—"Gourmet"	22	500-680
Ice Cream—Regular	16	300-360
Ice Cream—"Light"	10	220-260
Ice Cream—"FatFree"	—	200-240
Sorbet/Sherbet	—	180-240
Frozen Yogurt	—	180-280

Use low-fat versions of all dairy products. Check the information on labels routinely since there are wide varieties between different brands. Remember, "low-fat" does not always translate to "low calorie" because of the extra sugar added.

Day 39

Oil

Oils are fats mostly derived from plant sources and are liquid at room temperature. Examples are olive oil, corn oil, cottonseed oil, safflower oil, soybean oil, sunflower oil, and peanut oil. Oils are often used for frying.

Deep-fried foods, especially when battered or breaded, absorb considerable amounts of oil and should be avoided. **Instead of frying, steam, boil, poach, bake, broil, or barbecue.**

Day 40

Oil

Few fats and oils are composed exclusively of one type of the saturated, polyunsaturated, or monounsaturated fats. Most contain all three in some ratio, which determines the category in which fat is classified. Examples:

Oil	Saturated Percent	Monounsaturated Percent	Polyunsaturated Percent
Coconut	87	6	2
Corn	13	24	59
Olive	13	74	8
Safflower	9	12	75
Soybean	14	23	58
Sunflower	10	20	66

Avoid using oils that contain high levels of saturated fat. Choose oils rich in polyunsaturated fat and especially rich in monounsaturated fat, such as olive oil. Always use small amounts.

Day 41

Mind Power

Your mind has tremendous power. Make your mental power your best ally.

You are the ultimate authority. The determination to lose weight must come from you. Achieving your goal of a trim and fit body must be your decision.

Make slimming down a definite priority. Be fully committed to getting rid of the extra pounds.

Accept the responsibility of achieving your objective. **You are the one in charge. You are in control.** Learn to love and nurture yourself.

Day 42

Protein

An excess of animal protein is not only unnecessary but also harmful. It has been associated with an increased risk of developing obesity, heart disease and kidney problems.

One small serving (2-3 oz.) of animal protein per day is more than adequate to satisfy the protein requirements of an adult. Children, adolescents, and pregnant or lactating women need more, relative to their body weight.

Day 43

Protein

Avoid processed meats, such as bologna, salami, sausage, ham, and frankfurter, which usually contain too much fat and salt.

If you must have cold cuts, choose the leaner varieties such as sliced turkey breast, chicken breast, or smoked shaved turkey. For sandwiches, use only two or three slices of the cold cuts and one slice of lowfat cheese. Stuff the sandwich with lettuce, cucumbers, tomatoes, onions, and other favorite vegetables. Use pickles, herbs, spices and mustard generously.

Day 44

Behavior

You will not be able to fully enjoy even your most favorite foods, snacks, or desserts if you swallow them automatically, while you are distracted doing something else.

Make eating an event. Prepare your favorite gourmet dishes. Relish the delicacies for the flavor and quality, so you will not need the excessive quantity. **Pay attention to the colors, aroma, flavors, and texture of the food in your plate. Be conscious of every bite.** You will then thoroughly enjoy it and feel even more satisfied.

Day 45

Carbohydrates

Vegetables and fruit are among the most valuable foods that you can eat. These complex carbohydrates are essential for good health. They are **rich sources of minerals, vitamins, and fiber, are relatively low in calorie content**, come in a variety of delicious choices and are filling and satisfying because they provide ample bulk.

Compensate for the smaller amount of animal protein in your diet with generous servings of vegetables.

Choose fruit over rich, processed snacks, sweets and desserts at all times.

Day 46

Carbohydrates

Preparation methods of complex carbohydrates are crucial in maintaining their nutritional value. Batter frying vegetables or turning them into casseroles dripping with butter, creamy sauces, and cheese packs them with fat and calories, and turns them into health hazards. Serving fruit as desserts such as in pies, tarts, and shortcakes, places them in the category to be avoided.

Vegetables are best eaten raw, steamed, broiled, barbecued, or boiled, served with spices, balsamic vinegar or your favorite condiments.

Peaches, nectarines, apricots, kiwis, and mangos are just a few of the wide variety of delicious healthful treats.

Day 47

Carbohydrates

Brown rice, beans, cracked wheat, potatoes, whole grain breads, cereals, and pasta are considered to be mainstays of a healthy diet. Not only are these grain products and legumes low in fat and rich in vitamins and fiber, but they also are filling and satisfying.

Gradually rely more on these wholesome complex carbohydrates.

Use minimal amounts of fat or oil for cooking.

The creative use of herbs, spices, fresh lemon juice, vinegar, garlic, onion, and celery adds tremendous flavor and aroma to help reduce or eliminate the need for excessive fat.

Day 48

Paella

Rice with vegetables.

2 Tbsp olive oil
1 cup long-grain rice
2 1/2 cups no-fat chicken broth
1/2 cup string beans
1 can atrichoke hearts
1/2 cup frozen peas, thawed
1/2 cup water chestnuts
pinch black pepper
1 medium onion
1 carrot
1/2 red pepper
2 cloves garlic
1/2 tsp salt
1/2 cup mushrooms

Chop all vegetables and set aside. Heat the oil in a large pan, sauté onions until transparent. Add garlic, then rice and stir for one minute. Add chicken broth, string beans, carrots, red pepper and salt, let come to a boil. Simmer on low heat for twenty minutes. Add remaining ingredients, stir, and simmer covered until all liquid is absorbed. Let rest for fifteen minutes before serving.

(140-160 calories per cup.)

Day 49

Water

The adult human body consists of 60 to 70 percent water.

Water is essential for life. It is vital for the healthy physiological performance of the various organs and complex systems of the body.

Fluid is continuously lost through sweat, urine, breathing, and other processes. The delicate balance must be maintained by constantly replacing the water lost.

Drink water frequently. Eight glasses a day are recommended.

Day 50

Behavior

Television viewers seem to follow a certain routine during commercial breaks. They go looking for something to eat, not so much because of hunger, but simply for the lack of something to do to fill the gap.

Give it some thought. Break the pattern. Develop the new habit of substituting some form of physical activity or exercise for the snack. **During commercials get up and jog in place, do sit-ups or push-ups.** You will find these activities invigorating and refreshing.

Take up the challenge. Stretch your comfort zone!

Day 51

Food Portions

Reducing fat intake, even eliminating it completely, does not lead to weight loss when portion control is not in place. **Total number of calories consumed does count.**

You will not lose weight simply by replacing your chocolate chip cookies with cookies declaring zero fat content, if you eat too many of them.

Pasta is good but if you eat several servings at one sitting, you will gain weight, even if the spaghetti sauce contains no fat.

Control the amount you eat. Do not overeat.

Day 52

Calories

The food we eat provides the nutrients that the body processes into available sources of energy for all the physiological and developmental needs of the body, as well as the energy needed for physical activities.

The unit by which we measure the energy required to sustain our body, the energy we burn up while involved in physical activity, and the energy source contained in foods we eat is **the calorie.**

Day 53

Calories

Body movement and physical activity of all kinds use up energy over and above the energy needed at rest.

Within a range of plus or minus 400 calories, an adult man, depending on body size, may use around 1,600 calories a day at rest, 2,200 calories in the course of a day of ordinary activity, and 2,800 on a day of competitive sports and games.

Children need relatively more calories in proportion to their body weight and size.

Day 54

Calories

Depending on body size, within a range of plus or minus 400 calories, an adult woman may use around 1,300 calories a day at rest, 1,800 calories for a day of ordinary activity, and 2,300 for intensive activity.

Pregnant and lactating women need more than these estimated figures.

Athletes may need an additional 500 calories a day, depending on the specific training, the intensity, and the particular sports in which they are involved.

Day 55

Figure Out Your Average Daily Calorie Intake

Consult the table that lists the calorie content of some common foods at the end of this book. Refer to the labels on food packages that list the calories in the meals you eat.

Record all you eat and drink—meals, snacks, and drinks. Estimate the total daily amount you have eaten.

Keep records for a week and estimate the average daily amount of calories that you are currently consuming.

Day 56

Calories

The average American woman eats about 1,700 to 2,300 calories a day. An average man about 2,600 to 3,200. Because of variations in body size and metabolic rate, some maintain their weight at this level, others put on several pounds a year.

If you are maintaining your weight, to promote a weight loss of one pound per week, you should eat 500 fewer calories each day.

If you are putting on weight, in addition to reducing food consumption by 500 calories a day, you must start a program of significant physical activity to burn up the calories.

Day 57

Calories

A long-term menu plan of five hundred calories less than your usual daily total intake will steadily eliminate the extra pounds by a healthy one pound per week.

The easiest way to accomplish this is to reduce drastically the items with awfully high fat content, such as potato chips, french fries, cream, fatty meats, butter, fried foods, ice cream, candy bars, milk shakes, and regular sodas.

Keep a record of all you eat and drink.

Day 58

Calories

A preferable alternative to reducing calorie intake is a consistent increase in daily physical activity, which will burn up extra calories.

Thus instead of cutting down about 500 calories a day, it is far healthier to cut back around 300 calories a day and burn off the remaining roughly 200 calories or more with consistent regular physical activity.

Day 59

Physical Activity

To make the choice of a specific exercise routine, take the following into consideration:

—Do you prefer exercising alone or in a group? Is privacy important to you?
—Is this activity enjoyable for you?
—Will you do it on a regular basis?
—Is there a financial cost involved? Can you afford it?
—Does it fit your schedule?

Choose an activity with which you feel comfortable.

Day 60

Physical Activity

It is crucial to start any physical activity slowly and gradually. Do not start with a sudden dramatic change. Do not rush. It took years for your body to get out of shape; it will take time to get it to respond. The aim is to develop an exercise plan or activity that you can adhere to and enjoy for the rest of your life.

If you are still procrastinating, start by using the stairs instead of the elevator whenever possible.

Day 61

Walking

Walking is an enjoyable and uplifting experience that you can safely follow at any age throughout your life. It is also the easiest for people who are overweight or out of shape.

Awaken your enthusiasm for self-renewal and discover for yourself the joy of feeling fit. **Start by slow steady walking—indoor, outdoor, on your neighborhood school track or in the mall.**

Go ahead and do it. You owe it to yourself.

Day 62

Your Personal Commitment

Write down a clear statement of your determination to be trim and fit.

Identify the compelling reasons that initiated the turning point for seriously committing to this invigorating new lifestyle. Clarify your purpose and goal. **Believe you can achieve that goal. Record that you are committed to building a healthier future.**

Post this statement inside a kitchen cabinet door so you can refer to it whenever you need reinforcement, encouragement, and support.

Day 63

New Eating Habits

If your are routinely following a pattern of eating meals and snacks all over the house, it indicates that too many rooms and areas at home are associated with food and thus act as stimuli for eating. This mental association must be eliminated.

Select one specific place—such as the table in the kitchen or dining area—**in your living quarters and enjoy all meals, including snacks and beverages, sitting comfortably at that designated table.** This will help control impulsive eating.

Day 64

Behavior

To strengthen your resolve to eat only in one specific area, keep food and snacks in the kitchen and dining area, and eliminate food from the rest of the house. No cookies in the den, no candy in the living room, and certainly no crackers in the bedroom. It puts an end to helping yourself to a snack just because "it's there."

If you are hungry, go to your designated place, choose a healthy snack, sit down, enjoy every morsel, and feel good about yourself.

Day 65

Eat Slowly

Eating slowly allows the signals of gratification to reach your brain before you overeat. Please remember to always **e-a-t s-l-o-w-l-y.** Do not rush through a meal. Relax and linger over lunch and dinner. Think of it as a welcome break in your busy day. You will feel satisfied with less food.

An additional bonus of eating slowly is the increased enjoyment of food. You can concentrate on the color, texture, aroma, and flavor of the meal and thus enhance the pleasure of dining.

Day 66

Behavior

When you settle down for a long talk on the telephone, do you mindlessly reach for the cookie jar? Stop! Use your cordless phone and instead of sitting down, pace the floor while talking.

When you curl up in your favorite chair with a good book, do you munch on candy bars? Not any more! Sip a glass of water while you read.

If you decide to have a snack, put the book down, get off the phone, sit down at the table, and enjoy the snack.

Day 67

At Work

Plan ahead for the entire week. Have all the wholesome ingredients ready for your sandwiches and snacks.

Pack your lunch and take it to work. This allows you to plan ahead and prepare healthy, low-calorie, nutritious, and filling foods that are good for you, and help you lose or maintain your weight.

You will not have to rely on the calorie-laden fast foods that are the usual take-outs. You also eliminate luncheon outings and impulsive eating of fattening empty calories. You are in control.

Day 68

Compare

Take-out Foods	Calories
Cheeseburger	300-330
French Fries (large)	270-330
Milk Shake	330-380
Total calories	900-1,040
Suggestions	
Salad with grilled chicken no-oil dressing, or	200-250
Sandwich 1 oz. grilled chicken, lettuce, tomatoes, mustard	250-280
Low-calorie soda	0-10

Day 69

Eating Out

Plan ahead. Go for it!

Before you even get to the restaurant, before you pick up the tempting menu, plan what you intend to order. Exercise wise judgment based on the know-how you have gained and the new eating habits you have mastered. Your resolve will help you make wiser choices.

Let your companions know in advance that you are watching what you eat. Stay firm on your wholesome and healthful choices. Do not give in to their pressure. Set a great example, and earn the respect and admiration of your friends for your determination and discipline.

Day 70

Celebrations

Have fun!

Celebrating special occasions invariably evokes visions of drinking and eating. This attitude needs to be reevaluated and revised. “Celebrating” should not automatically translate into drinking and overindulging.

Instead of celebrating the occasion in a restaurant, **shift the focus to an evening at the theater. Take in the new play in town.**

Better still, go somewhere you can dance, and celebrate while burning calories!

Day 71

Keep Records

Stick to it!

Monitoring your food intake and activity levels will help increase your awareness of self-defeating eating habits. As you identify the destructive habits that have caused your weight problem, you will be able to replace them with healthy, constructive attitudes about food and eating.

Self-monitoring leads to self-mastery and self-control. Keep records of the food that you eat and your physical activities.

Identify self-defeating habits and work on them.

Day 72

Rewards

Hurray for you!

Ladies! Update and improve your makeup to highlight your beauty assets and to bring out your best features. You may wish to consult a beautician at your favorite department store cosmetic counter.

Gentlemen! Wear brighter, bolder ties. Dress well!

You will be showered with compliments from family, colleagues, and friends for your progress and accomplishment. Your sense of achievement and pride will give you renewed determination and drive.

Day 73

Reflections

People are motivated to lose weight for a variety of reasons.

For some, the triggering incident might be a peek at a recent photograph or videotape of themselves. For others, anticipation of a dreaded birthday may act as a wake-up call. Some suddenly face serious medical problems, such as cardiovascular disease, that necessitates weight loss and exercise for health reasons.

Whatever the case, put it to good use and strengthen your commitment to achieve your goal.

Persistence is the key!

Day 74

Reinforcement

Inform your family, friends, and colleagues of your commitment to a healthier lifestyle and enlist their help. Ask them to support your choices of healthier food and not to offer you tempting alternatives, second helpings, fattening treats, or excuses to indulge "just this once" or to make an exception because of "this special occasion."

"Special occasions" and "exceptions" should be your decision, not theirs.

Let them know that you will appreciate it if they do not bring you sweet treats as a gift.

Day 75

Goals

Set realistic goals. Consider your gender, age, and inherited general body build while setting your goal.

If you are in your forties or beyond, it would be unrealistic for you to decide to get back to your weight in your late teens or early twenties. At a younger age, your metabolism and physiology were on an entirely different level, and you were much more active—you probably were participating in one of the team sports or track teams. Do not get unreasonably ambitious.

Day 76

Food Preparaiton

The correct method of food preparation is crucial for fat content and calories:
Compare:

Food	Average Calories
Baked potato, average, plain	100
Baked potato, 2 tbsp. butter	300
Same potato, served as hash-brown	700
Same potato, served as french fries	800

The plain potato contains all the wonderful nutrients you need, without the added burden of the fat and the calories. Top the potato with spices, herbs, condiments, and vegetables sautéed in chicken broth.

Try low-fat or non-fat varieties of sour cream.

Day 77

Salad Dressings

Just three tablespoons of dressing added to your innocent "healthful" salad will turn it into a source of oil and calories by adding anywhere from 190 to 250 calories.

—Reduce the amount of dressing you use.
—Try the nonfat dressings.
—Prepare your own with fresh lemon juice, balsamic vinegar, garlic, mustard, herbs, spices, and a touch of olive oil.

Day 78

Mayonnaise

Just one tablespoon of mayonnaise in your regular sandwich adds an unnecessary 100 calories to your daily lunch total. That adds up to (365 days x 100 cal/day) 36,500 calories a year, which translates into an additional ten pounds of fat possibly sneaking in on you.

Enrich your sandwiches with generous helpings of lettuce, tomatoes, cucumbers, and other favorite vegetables. Use spices, herbs, and mustard to add flavor and aroma.

Day 79

Low-fat Cooking Tips

Trim off all visible fat from meat or fowl before cooking.

Remove the skin from fowl, since the skin is almost all fat. When broiling or roasting, you can leave the skin on to prevent drying out, but discard before eating.

Broil, bake, or barbecue meat, poultry, and fish instead of frying.

Day 80

Plan Ahead

Planning your meals the day before prepares you mentally for the changes in your diet and makes it much easier to follow your new dietary guidelines.

Based on the information gained over previous weeks, plan the menu for the next day and jot it down. Have the items available. At mealtime, you will be programmed to reach for the foods that you had planned to eat.

Day 81

Protein

Each gram of pure protein contributes four calories, exactly the same as starch or any other carbohydrate. It is important to remember that most of the protein that you consume comes from animal flesh, which contains considerable amounts of fat. At nine calories per gram, the fat itself increases the total calorie count to much more than is estimated by the weight of the serving of meat as protein.

Choose small portions and lean cuts of meat.

Day 82

Fish

For shedding pounds and even beyond concerns of weight loss, one of the most important health habits to develop is to replace beef with fish as often as possible, provided the fish is not fried, batter-fried, or drenched in butter sauce. Skip the tartar sauce, use generous amounts of fresh lemon juice and spices.

The least fatty fish are cod, flounder, sole, haddock, and halibut. Salmon, mackerel, and swordfish have a higher fat content.

Day 83

Protein

Ideally, meat and poultry should be used as condiments to add flavor and protein enrichment to other dishes.

Instead of serving a huge steak or large chunks of chicken and turkey, slice, cube, or sliver the enormous servings, combine with generous amounts of vegetables, legumes, or grains and create a delightful salad, a flavorful soup, an aromatic stew or a delicious casserole that provides balanced nutrition.

Meat and poultry can also be added to salads.

Day 84

Protein

A meal does not have to contain any animal flesh at all. Low-fat or fat-free milk, cheese, or egg whites enhance the protein content of a starch, legume, or vegetable dish.

You might be pleasantly surprised to know that **the healthiest food sources for protein are grains, roots, seeds, legumes, and vegetables in unrefined, minimally processed form.** Good examples are various kinds of beans, peas, seeds, lentils, chickpeas, soybeans, and nuts.

Day 85

Vegetable Chili

A meal in itself

- 1 28-oz can crushed tomatoes
- 1 14-oz can low-fat chicken broth
- 1 onion
- 2 carrots
- 3 cloves garlic
- 1 can red kidney beans
- 1 can pinto beans
- 1 can white beans
- 1 can chick peas
- 1 can corn kernels
- 2 stalks celery
- 1 chili pepper
- 1/2 red pepper
- 1/4 cup parsley
- 1/2 tsp oregano
- 1/2 tsp salt
- 1/4 tsp cumin
- 1/2 tsp chili powder

Chop all vegetables. Drain all cans.

In a large pot, combine tomatoes and chicken broth. Add all chopped fresh vegetables and spices. Bring to a boil. Simmer for ten minutes, stirring occasionally. Add drained beans and corn. Stir. Bring to a boil. Turn heat off. Adjust seasonings.

(160-180 calories per cup. Generous protein, negligible fat).

Day 86

To Strengthen My Resolve

Advantages of Losing Weight.

—I will be healthier and more energetic.
—I will wear more stylish clothes.
—My blood pressure will be lower.
—I will be able to walk without getting out of breath.
—I will participate in sports activities.
—I will be more confident and outgoing.
—I will be very proud of myself.

Day 87

The Potato

One of the most maligned food items is the **potato**. It is considered a starchy source of high calories, but in truth it is a rich, low-calorie source of vitamins, minerals, and fiber. A medium sized potato, about five ounces, baked, boiled, or steamed, contributes only 100 calories.

Needless to say, this nutritious food is abundant, inexpensive, and very versatile. Eat it baked, in its natural, unadulterated form, with non-fat toppings.

Day 88

Bread

Let bread occupy its rightful place as an important and healthy component of your daily diet. It is ideally suited to your aim of reducing fat and calories. Unfortunately, fad diets generally shun bread as a fattening and worthless food, contributing nothing but calories.

The fact is that bread, especially whole-grain bread, multi-grain bread, bran and sprouted-wheat bread, is low in fat, relatively low in calories, but high in fiber content. What's more, it is filling, satisfies hunger, and is inexpensive.

Eliminate from your diet most of the rich, fatty foods, and substitute with whole-grain bread.

Day 89

Sugar

Sugar is a highly refined food stripped of its fiber and nutritional components; it lacks vitamins, minerals, and fiber, and offers nothing but empty calories.

Sugar is consumed in enormous quantities hidden in soft drinks, milk shakes, candy, chocolate, cakes, cookies, ice cream, and sugar-coated cereals. It adds substantial calories to food.

The excess sugar consumed, including honey, brown sugar, molasses and syrup, is stored by the body as fat and results in obesity. Gradually reduce the use of sugar to the absolute minimum.

Say good-bye to sugar! And smile!

Day 90

Reflections

Motivation to lose weight often relates to changes in life situations, such as divorce, a new job, a career change, a move to a new environment and new social circle. It may be the result of personal maturity and growth, changes in values, or a medical problem that forces a reevaluation of priorities.

Whatever the reason, seize the opportunity, put it to good use. Make losing weight a priority. Believe you can achieve this worthwhile goal. Take charge of your life. You deserve the best!

Day 91

Keep Records

Write it down!

—Use your pocket calendar.
—Keep a running record of your calorie intake and add total calories for the day.
—Mark down the type of physical activity and the duration.
—Record behavioral triumphs.
—Jot down your weight once a week.

Lack of time is not an excuse. We find time for things that are important to us.

Day 92

Keeping Records

Keeping track of calories helps you develop an awareness of the vast difference of calorie content of the many different foods available to you. It will help you distinguish between the healthy, low-calorie desirable foods that you should concentrate on, and the fatty, calorie-laden health hazards that you should avoid. Monitoring leads you to making the right choices and helps you stay within the range of calories you have planned.

Day 93

Preparing Meals

If you are in charge of preparing the meals for the entire family, you can:

—Prepare two separate dishes, using your favorite low-fat recipes for yourself.
—Reduce the amount of fat in your regular recipes for everyone's advantage.
—Separate your portion before you add the butter, oil, or cream to the food.
—Broil or bake your portion instead of frying, if they still insist on fried foods.
—Have a huge salad with fat-free dressing, and only a small helping of the family's food.

Day 94

Solid Fillers

Develop the habit of eating generous helpings of "solid fillers." These are the nutritious foods that are low in calories but provide abundant amounts of bulk and fiber to help you feel satisfied with less calories. Examples are celery, lettuce, carrots, cucumbers, broccoli, cauliflower, green and red peppers, grapefruit, or any favorite vegetable or fruit—all perfectly healthy foods.

A salad with low-fat dressing is the perfect complement to any lunch or dinner.

Day 95

Calories

A pound of fat is equivalent to 3,500 calories of energy. Therefore, **to lose an average of one pound a week, you should burn up 3,500 calories more than the calories you eat in one week. That translates into cutting down your total daily intake of calories by an average of 500 and simultaneously increasing your workout to use up more calories.**

The body draws on fat stores for energy when it is unable to get the calories from food intake and thus reduces fat deposits.

Day 96

Calories

Total calorie intake does make a difference. So does calorie expenditure.

Weight loss can be achieved by cutting back on calories consumed and by burning up more calories with increased levels of exercise.

The most desirable way to achieve healthy weight loss is to develop a lifestyle that includes a combination of reduced calorie intake and increased physical activity levels.

It is never too late to implement the changes that are going to lead you to achieve your goals. Do what is right.

Day 97

Physical Activity

Physical activity uses up calories to provide the energy required by the exercise. Action burns up body fat when the calorie intake is limited.

Activity	Calories Used Per Hour
Swimming, continuous, slow	260-360
Tennis, doubles	300-360
Tennis, singles	420-480
Walking, 3 mph	240-300
Walking, 5 mph	420-540
Jogging, 5 mph	500-600
Swimming, competitive	400-500

Which will it be?

Day 98

Physical Activity

If you are already involved in a reasonable amount of exercise, strive to increase your current activities, gradually raising the frequency and extending the duration of your workout. **Aim at exercising half an hour a day, at least three times a week.** Once you have established a steady exercise routine, work on increasing the intensity of the activity.

Put your heart and soul into what you do!

Day 99

Walking

Walking does not require membership in any club or sports facility. You can walk almost anytime, anywhere at no cost to you. Walking requires no special equipment or clothing other than a pair of comfortable walking shoes. It can be done alone, with a companion or in a group, indoors or outdoors.

Everyone can walk. No special talent, skill, or training is required. The risk of injury is low with walking since it is less stressful to weight-bearing joints.

Take up walking and go at it with enthusiasm and excitement. Just do it!

Day 100

Walking

Lack of time is not a valid reason for not exercising; it is just an excuse. Since physical activity makes you feel more energetic and helps you lose weight, you owe it to yourself to set aside some time, at least every other day, to take care of your own health. Put it high up on your priority list.

Let today mark the beginning of your rejuvenation! Start by walking ten minutes every other day at a convenient time.

Gradually increase it to twenty, then thirty minutes. Later on, work towards a faster pace until you walk a brisk half-hour.

Day 101

Water

Following strenuous physical activity, you will be thirsty, indicating your body's physiological need to replace fluid and electrolyte loss through perspiration.

Make sure you drink plenty of water, or non-caloric fluids such as club soda or diet drinks to compensate for the body fluids lost during workout.

Carry bottled water with you to sip during outdoor workouts, especially on warm, sunny days.

Day 102

Food Fiber

Food fiber is that part of plants, roots, seeds, vegetables, and fruit that our alimentary system cannot digest or absorb. Found in abundance in a highly unrefined complex carbohydrate diet, it increases the volume of the food in your stomach and promotes a feeling of fullness, thus satisfying hunger with lower total calorie intake.

Eat lots of salads, vegetables, legumes, and fruit.

Day 103

Liquids

In addition to water, a variety of other beverages, such as milk, coffee, tea, soft drinks, fruit juices, and vegetable juices, contribute fluid too. However:

Although delicious and rich in vitamins, fruit juices can add a lot of unwanted calories. Drink them conservatively.

Along with great nutrition, milk adds unnecessary fat. Drink only skim or fat-free milk.

Soft drinks are often laden with sugar, calories, caffeine, and artificial sweeteners. Sparkling water, seltzer water, and mineral water would be the ideal replacements.

Day 104

Alcohol

From the perspective of nutrition and calories alone, alcohol has practically no nutritive value—just empty calories similar to sugar. But those calories are considerable:

Alcoholic Beverage	Amount	Calories
Distilled spirits: gin, rum, vodka, whisky	1 jigger	100-125
Liqueurs	1 oz	80-100
Sherry	4 oz	160-200
Vermouth	4 oz	120-190
Wines	4 oz	100-115
Beer, light, regular	12 oz	105-155

Day 105

Alcohol

Alcoholic beverages add a lot of calories, for zero nutritional returns. On the contrary, the harmful effects of excessive alcohol consumption are well documented.

There is new evidence that one drink a day might help lower the rate of heart disease.

Decrease alcohol consumption to the bare minimum of one drink a day and use those calories to eat a balanced, nutritious, and filling meal instead.

Day 106

Wine

Recent studies have shown the beneficial effects of wine. These studies were based on the observation that the French, who drink wine routinely with their meals, have lower incidences of cardiovascular problems, even though they consume liberal amounts of fat contained in their creamy sauces and cheeses.

It might be advisable to have a glass of red wine occasionally with dinner. **The benefits seem to outweigh the added calories.**

Day 107

Grape Juice

Further investigation of the beneficial effects of a glass of red wine indicates that the effective factors are the antioxidants found in the skin of red grapes.

Hence, eating red grapes or drinking purple grape juice will have similar desirable benefits for the cardiovascular system and is recommended as a good alternative to wine, especially for those who choose not to consume alcohol.

Day 108

Reinforcement

Long-term clinical studies have shown that people who lost considerable amounts of weight, and maintained the reduced weight for decades, did so by following the same basic principles and tips that this guide recommends.

You too can master the same essential principles. With consistent, gradual changes, you can develop a new way of living where you:

—Take charge of your life.
—Develop healthy attitudes and habits regarding food and eating.
—Modify the menus and recipes you use.
—Make wiser food choices.
—Adopt an active, energetic lifestyle.

Day 109

Goal

Set an achievable goal. Do not put yourself in a situation in which you decide to lose too many pounds in too short a time, making it impossible to accomplish. That is counterproductive.

Depending on how overweight you are, plan to drop one or two pounds per week, and figure out your short-term and long-term goals accordingly. Your success will encourage you and motivate you to go on.

You can achieve it!

Day 110

Persistence Is the Key

It is helpful to learn from people who have mastered weight loss and weight maintenance—those who are in control of their eating habits and lifestyle.

You will discover that they did so by starting again every time they had a setback, by getting back on track every time they veered off their healthy decision, by renewing their commitments every time their discipline and resolve weakened.

Positive attitude, effective action, and single-minded persistence work wonders.

Keep up the good work!

Day 111

Appetite

Eating is often initiated by the proximity or availability of food. You find yourself eating because:

—The food is right there.
—It is time to eat.
—It is all included and paid for.
—It is free; you are an invited guest.
—It was especially prepared for you.

These situations have nothing to do with the need for nutrition. The proximity, smell, and visibility of food stimulate appetite, regardless of the fact that you are not hungry. Be alert to this distinction.

Do you really need that food? If not, save it and eat part of it at another meal.

Day 112

Hunger

Hunger results from the physiological need of the body for nourishment. The hungry person feels "stomach cramps" and "hunger pangs," indicating the need for a source of energy.

Hunger is distinctly different from emotional cravings. It signals the body's legitimate need for nutrition.

Make a clear distinction between appetite and hunger. Where hunger is indicated, satisfy the need with healthy choices of food.

Enjoy!

Day 113

Hunger

As newborns, food was our first tranquilizer. As infants, we were fed when we cried. As children, we were calmed with sweets when we scraped our knee. Candy bars were rewards when we "were good." As a result, sweets and dessert have been associated with pleasure and reward—not with hunger or need.

As adults, we often turn to food or sweets when feeling sad or generally "low."

Note your feelings when you are reaching for a snack. Are you hungry? Are you looking for an emotional lift? If you are truly hungry, then by all means enjoy a healthy snack.

Day 114

Behavior

To reinforce your decision of eating only in the one place to be associated with eating, **choose a "Designated Place" different from your usual seat at the table.** This will make you more aware of your commitment and more receptive to change. Your chosen "Designated Place" could be across the table from your former seat.

The same rule of designating only one place for eating applies for the office as well.

Day 115

Eat Slowly

Interesting. . . . You never realized how fast you ate. . . .

An easy and effective way to slow down eating is the practice of **putting down the fork between every morsel** during your meal. Take small morsels, place the fork down, chew well, and swallow each mouthful of food before picking up the fork again for another morsel.

Take time. Relax and relish your food.

Day 116

At Work

For "coffee breaks" with coworkers, bring along your own low-calorie snacks, such as non-fat yogurt, fat-free pretzels, an apple, an orange, or a banana, and forego the usual doughnuts and pastries.

You might be satisfied with just a cup of tea. The break is meant to offer you a refreshing change from the routine, a chance to rest, and an opportunity to socialize.

Eating Out

Do not hesitate to make inquiries about the contents of a specific menu item before you order:

—Is the soup made with cream?
—Does this dish have cheese in it?
—How is the fish prepared? Is it fried?

Request that they kindly:

—Bake, broil, or barbecue the fish without any butter or oil.
—Serve your vegetables steamed without any butter or sauces.
—Not add any dressing to your salad, but bring some lemon, olive oil, mustard, or balsamic vinegar on the side.

Day 118

Celebrating

If you have a special celebration coming up, go all out and splurge. **But plan to do so ahead of time.**

When you plan to indulge, you are very much in control. You can enjoy the special treat and then resume your new eating habits.

Praise yourself for being in charge and for the progress you have made. Give yourself recognition for your gradual weight loss.

Day 119

Buying Food

Shop for groceries when you are not hungry—when you are not craving to eat everything in sight.

It is easier for you to avoid temptation, adhere to your prepared list of groceries, and to stick to the healthy choices you have made, when you're not ravenous.

Day 120

Storing Food

Eliminate from your living quarters and place of employment all the foods that you have decided not to eat. Get rid of items you have trouble resisting. Do not keep around snacks, like candy bars, pastries, ice cream, and potato chips that tempt you. You can't be lured in a moment of weakness by snacks that are not available.

Day 121

Rewards

You are doing great!

Reward yourself with new clothes. Buy a new dress, a pair of pants, or a suit in a smaller size. Be bold. Choose the brighter colors and fashionable styles that you have been avoiding.

The positive feedback from the people around you will strengthen your transfer of gratification from food to feeling good about yourself, and will give you renewed motivation.

Stand up tall and proud.

Day 122

Keep Busy

People who have few interests are liable to eat more out of boredom than for any other reason. We resort to mindless nibbling for lack of interesting and rewarding preoccupation, purpose, and direction.

Keep busy. Volunteer your services to one of the worthwhile projects in your community.

Take up a hobby that interests you. It could be woodwork, furniture refinishing, sewing, quilting, knitting, sketching, painting, or gardening. New activities will open up new horizons, offer a chance to make new friends, and help decrease your preoccupation with food.

Day 123

Mistakes Are Learning Experiences

An occasional lapse is simply a normal mistake, not evidence of weakness, failure, or lack of will power. After an unintentional binge, take some time to think about what happened. Figure out why it happened—what precipitated it.

Use the insight gained from this experience to handle urges better in the future. Make a mental note to help you control a similar situation the next time it comes up. Go back on schedule and pick up where you left off.

Be good to yourself.

Day 124

Review

Review the tips presented so far. Mark the pages of the information, guidelines, and suggestions that you find especially helpful or relevant. Write down your own secrets of success. Refer to them occasionally and practice them faithfully.

Repetition and reinforcement help develop new good habits. Strengthen your resolve and energize yourself by periodically reviewing those specific pages.

Keep up the good work!

Day 125

Fat

Each gram of fat and oil that you consume adds 9 calories to the total, in contrast to 4 calories per gram of proteins and 4 calories per gram of carbohydrates. Thus ounce per ounce, fats and oils supply more than twice as many calories as do carbohydrates or proteins.

Select foods that are low in fat. You will be able to eat the same quantity of food, but take in less calories. For example:

One pound of	Fat Grams	Calories
Lean ground beef	75-85	1150-1230
Chicken (no skin)	16-40	760-870
Flounder (no skin)	**6-10**	**310-360**

Day 126

Fat

An ounce of fat has approximately 270 calories, while an ounce of either pure protein or carbohydrate has just 120.

Thus, when you cut back on fat, you get to eat a much larger portion of low-fat or fat-free food for any given calorie level; you feel fuller and more satisfied.

For 240 calories, you can eat:

Either	Or
3 oz french fries	12 oz of baked potatoes
2 oz cheddar cheese	10 oz lean steamed fish
1 1/2 oz potato chips	1 lb of apples

For your health, your future, your life, make the smarter choices.

Day 127

Cholesterol

Cholesterol is a waxy fat that is vital for normal physiologic function. There is no dietary requirement for cholesterol, however, because the body can synthesize what it needs.

Excess blood cholesterol can be life-threatening, forming plaque on artery walls, restricting the flow of oxygen-carrying blood to vital organs, and causing high blood pressure, stroke, or heart problems.

Reduce the intake of dietary cholesterol by avoiding foods that contain high levels of cholesterol, such as animal fat, bacon, egg yolk, and cheese. Read the labels of packaged foods.

Day 128

Cholesterol

Oils, which come mostly from plant sources, contain no cholesterol and consist mainly of mono-unsaturated and poly-unsaturated fats. Of these, olive oil even helps reduce blood cholesterol levels.

Replace saturated fat in your diet with small amounts of polyunsaturated fat. Use vegetable oil instead of butter.

Where taste will allow, use olive oil instead of the other vegetable oils that your recipes call for.

Day 129

Low-fat Cooking Tips

—Poach poultry or fish in low-fat chicken broth, tomato juice, or water seasoned with spices and herbs, lemon juice, or wine.
—Steam vegetables and fish. Season with spices, lemon juice, and herbs.
—Use nonstick pots and pans for sautéed vegetables. Brush on a light coating of oil, or spray on non-stick vegetable oil.

Day 130

Behavior

Time for a change.

When you return home, do you automatically look for something to eat? Do you find yourself heading to the refrigerator, reaching for a snack, regardless of the fact that you just came back from a dinner engagement?

Give up the bad habit; change the old pattern. Avoid the kitchen completely. Check your mail, read the newspaper, socialize with loved ones.

If you end up strolling in the kitchen, have a glass of water.

Day 131

Protein

Red meat is not at all necessary as a source of protein. Chicken, turkey, and fish are excellent sources of protein, and are generally lower in fat and calories.

4 oz Porterhouse steak, broiled	520 calories
4 oz Porterhouse steak fat trimmed, broiled	260 calories
4 oz chicken, broiled, no skin	190 calories

Whenever possible, choose chicken over beef, **provided it is not fried, and the fat and skin are not consumed.**

Day 132

Protein

As a general rule, it would be wise to use only half of the amount of meat indicated in recipes for beef casseroles, beef stews, and dishes using ground beef. Replace the balance with a larger amount of the vegetables, legumes, or grains.

As an alternative, double the vegetables, legumes, and grains of the recipes while keeping the amount of beef the same.

Day 133

Eggs

Eggs contain only about 80 calories each. Preparation methods, however, will change the total calorie contribution of an egg served for breakfast. The calories double or triple if an egg is fried in generous amounts of butter or fat. Served with bacon, sausages, or hash browns, the calorie count soars dramatically.

Replace fried eggs with poached, soft-boiled, or hard-boiled eggs, accompanied by plain whole-wheat bread or an English muffin.

Day 134

Goals

Believe in yourself. You deserve the best.

People who believe in themselves have an easier time achieving their goals. Those who believe they can achieve what they have set out to do focus better, follow their decisions and commitments with more persistence, and get better results.

Believe in yourself firmly. Positive affirmations boost your ego and empowering thoughts affirm your belief in yourself.

Keep going. You're doing great!

Day 135

Legumes

Legumes, such as dried beans, peas, chickpeas, lentils, and soybeans are among the most nutritious foods at our disposal. They are widely available and inexpensive.

Legumes contain generous amounts of high quality proteins, lots of fiber, abundant complex carbohydrates, lots of vitamins and minerals. They are cholesterol-free, and the small amount of fat in them is largely the desirable polyunsaturated kind.

Take charge. Do what's good for you.

Day 136

Beans

Few other foods can provide the nutritional value of beans and the variety of tastes, colors, and textures that beans offer. They are versatile and can be used in dips, salads, soups, sandwiches, spreads, and snacks as well as main dishes.

Used in combination with grains, such as rice, cracked wheat, oats, corn, or milk, these legumes also provide complete protein nutrition.

Make the choices that will help you look good and feel good.

Day 137

Soybeans

The soybean stands out among the family of beans as a rich source of plant protein. It is available as roasted nuts, or in the pods among the frozen vegetables, to be boiled, shelled, and enjoyed.

Soybean is used as the main ingredient for the preparation of various products, such as soy milk and tofu. The latter is the non-dairy counterpart of cheese. It is high in protein, has no cholesterol, and the fat it contains is unsaturated.

Try soy milk and experiment with tofu in salads, stews, and casseroles. Give it a try!

Day 138

Protein

Expensive steaks in restaurants are usually well marbled with fat. As a result they actually have less protein per pound than leaner cuts of beef. About half of the calories in marbled or fatty meat come from the fat. We are consuming a lot of unnecessary extra calories and a lot of undesirable saturated fat and cholesterol if we insist on getting our protein from beef.

Experiment with beans, especially soybeans, as healthy low-calorie, cholesterol-free sources of protein.

Day 139

The Potato

Baked potatoes taste great topped with vegetables lightly sautéed in their own juices. Onions, tomatoes, mushrooms, green peppers, red peppers, broccoli, and other vegetables sautéed in chicken broth make delicious toppings as well. Yogurt can be a good alternative.

Sweet potatoes and yams baked in the oven are so rich in flavor that they can be enjoyed as is, without any additions or toppings.

Day 140

Ratatouille

Eggplant and Zucchini Casserole

1 eggplant	2 zucchinis
1 red pepper	1 large onion
3 cloves garlic	1 tsp salt
1 can chick peas	1 tsp oregano
3 tbsp vinegar	1/4 tsp thyme
2 tbsp olive oil	pinch of cayenne
1 can crushed tomatoes	1/2 cup water

Chop all vegetables coarsely.

Heat the olive oil in a large pot. Add onion and sauté; add garlic, eggplant, zucchini, pepper, vinegar, and stir to coat. Add remaining ingredients and spices. Bring to a boil. Cover and simmer for one hour. Uncover and simmer fifteen minutes more to reduce liquid. Adjust seasonings.

Serve with rice or as a side dish. Enjoy! Note: Can be served as a topping for baked potatoes too.

120-140 calories and 3 grams of fat per cup.

Day 141

Bread

In a misguided effort to lower consumption of calories, well-meaning people often discard the two slices of bread from their sandwich and eat the fatty half-inch-thick cold cuts, cheese, and mayonnaise, which contribute anywhere between 400 to 500 calories, and too much fat. Together with the potato chips and large soft drink, the total could add up to 900 calories!

In contrast, two slices of whole grain bread, two or three slices of the cold cuts, and generous amounts of tomatoes, lettuce, and spiced mustard amount to no more than 300 calories. Eliminate the mayonnaise and the chips, and do not "waste" calories on soft drinks.

Day 142

Sugar

The more sugar you use, the more you will crave it. **Gradually reduce the amount of sugar you add to your coffee and tea.** It is a learned habit that can be changed over time. Your taste buds will adjust and you will be satisfied with much less.

It will take time to clear the excess sugar from your system, but you will be delighted to have eliminated the sugar dependency and the craving for sweet, high-caloric snacks.

Day 143

Calories

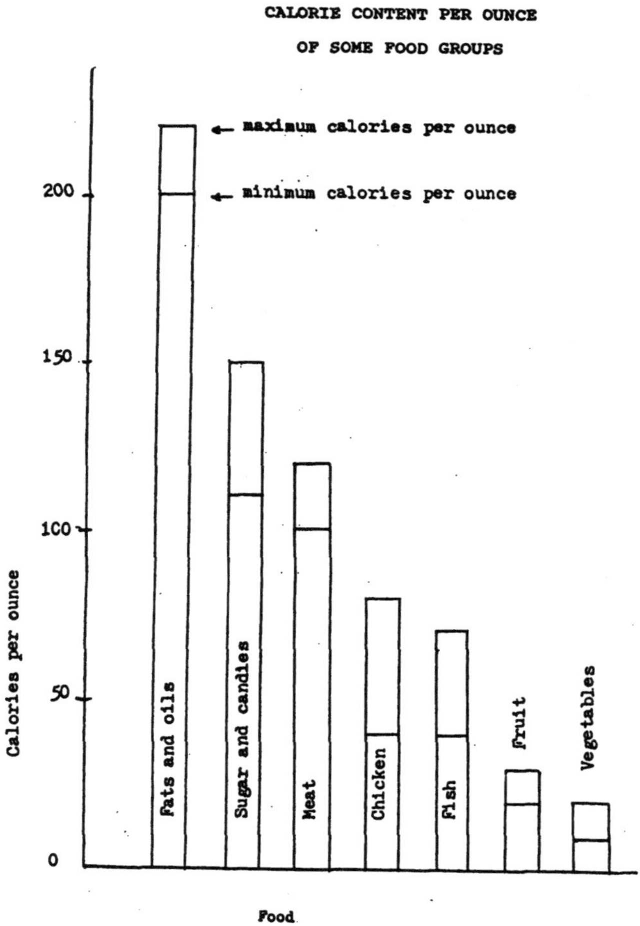

Day 144

In Summary

Aim at eating more of the produce that nature has provided for us from the very beginning; foods that have been available over the millennia of the development of the human race; foods that our digestive and metabolic systems evolved to accommodate. Eat:

More	Less
Vegetables	Fat, oil, butter
Fruit	Processed foods
Whole grain cereal, bread, pasta	Sweets, alcohol
Legumes	Pork
Fish, fowl	Beef

Day 145

Compare:

1 lb. of	Average Calorie Content
Cabbage, trimmed	110
Cauliflower, raw, flowerets	120
Broccoli, raw, trimmed	145
Carrots	190
Potatoes, baked	325
Sweet potatoes, baked	500
Chicken, roasted, no skin	800
Porterhouse steak, lean, broiled no bone	1,000
Cheddar Cheese	1,800

Be selective and discriminating with your food choices.

Day 146

Creamy Carrot Soup

A delicious "cream soup" without any cream or butter! A real treat.

2 14-oz cans fat-free chicken broth
2 potatoes, peeled, cut in chunks
8-10 carrots peeled, cut coarsely
1 large onion, cut coarsely
2 stalks celery, cut in chunks
2 cloves garlic
1 teaspoon salt
1 cup water
Fresh ground black pepper

In a large pot, combine all ingredients, except for the black pepper. Bring to a boil. Simmer until vegetables are tender. Purée in blender or food processor. Add black pepper. Adjust salt to taste. Adjust consistency with more water if necessary. Serve warm with whole wheat crackers.

80-100 calories per cup.

Note: Enjoy pea soup too by replacing the carrots with a large package of frozen peas.

Day 147

Fiber

The typical American diet, which relies heavily on processed and refined foods and snacks, does not provide enough fiber. To increase fiber content, include plenty of whole-grain bread, cereals, legumes, vegetables, and fruit in your diet.

Because of their natural high-fiber content, complex carbohydrates require more chewing; slow down eating, and as a result discourage overeating too.

Day 148

Keep Records

Keeping a weight-control journal is essential for success. It is a great tool for monitoring your progress. It will provide a running record of your daily total calorie intake, your decreasing weight, your newly acquired healthy eating habits, and exercise routines.

Based on the total calories consumed during the day, you can make an informed decision as to whether you should have that extra snack after dinner or not.

If you are not keeping a journal, start one today. If you are recording, keep up the good work.

Day 149

Calories

Think of a daily calorie limit in terms of a budget, like your monthly expense budget. Just as you differentiate between less costly and more expensive items and tailor your expenditure based on your finances, **choose what you eat and how much of it you eat, to stay within your self-allotted "budget of calories."**

Eliminate foods that "cost too many calories" and eat generous helpings of the "inexpensive, low-calorie" items. Learn how to get the most amount of bulk for your total daily budget of calories. **"Spend" your calories wisely.**

Day 150

Calories

Spread out your calorie intake over the entire day. Example:

	Women	Men
Breakfast	200	300
Lunch	350	450
Dinner	600	750
Snack	100	150
Total Calories	1250	1650

Do not skip meals and then end up eating all your calories in one large meal.

Day 151

Calories

To lose weight, energy burned up must exceed food intake so that the body will use or burn its excess fat reserve to make up the difference between "food income" and "energy expenditure."

Since the body is a complex, living wonder geared for survival, many other factors come into play. Thus it is not a simple, straightforward, mathematical relationship.

Develop the good habit of satisfying your diet and energy needs without overeating.

Day 152

Candy Bars

Candy bars pack too much fat and calories.

Candy bar (in ounces)	Calories	Total fat
3 Musketeers (2.1)	260	8
Milky Way (2.1)	270	10
Snickers (2.1)	280	14
Nestle's Butterfinger (2.1)	270	11
Kit Kat (1.5)	220	11
Kit Kat (3.4)	500	26
M&M's (1.7)	270	10
M&M's (5.6)	800	34

Chocolate lovers, beware!

Day 153

Aerobic Dancing

If you prefer working out in group settings, you can sign up for aerobic exercises and dance classes offered at health clubs and community centers. The scheduled sessions help re-enforce your commitment and insure your participation. In addition to group interaction, these centers offer a variety of exercises and lively music.

Join the low-impact workouts, in which one foot is always on the ground, to eliminate lower back pain, and injury to knees and other joints.

If you are happy working out by yourself, get a basic beginners aerobics videotape.

Day 154

Walking

Walking is a natural activity, can be practiced at any time and any place, does not need partners or teammates, does not require expensive equipment and helps:

—Burn off calories
—Burn off fat
—Reduce weight
—Increase muscle tone
—Raise the basal metabolic rate
—Suppress appetite
—Improve blood circulation
—Improve heart function
—Improve general fitness

Day 155

Walking

Even if you have a busy schedule, you can incorporate walking in your daily routine:

If you live within walking distance from your work, make it a habit to walk to work and back every day.

If you drive to work, find free or less expensive parking a few blocks away and walk the distance both ways.

Take a half-hour walk during your lunch break.

While watching television, jog in place for the duration of a half-hour program.

Day 156

Goal

Set a healthy goal. It is often better to set health, improved eating habits, and physical activity as your goal rather than a predetermined number on the scale. The focus should be on healthy lifestyle changes.

The weight problem is an indication of the underlying risky lifestyle. Improved eating behavior, food choices, and activity levels result in a better quality of life, which in turn results in weight loss.

Day 157

Be Persistent

Remember that weight control is an ongoing process. It entails a lifelong commitment to giving up old bad habits and replacing them with new healthy behavior. It requires discontinuing self-defeating practices and adopting positive attitudes.

Remember also that losing weight is a slow process. Just as you gained the weight gradually, you will shed it just as slowly, to make it permanent.

Stick with it! Dwell on your victories. Give yourself recognition for your achievements.

Day 158

Hunger

Eating can sometimes be initiated by environmental factors.

You are at a ball game and “everyone else” is eating and drinking. The general atmosphere, the social setting, and longstanding feelings and habits drive you to eat mindlessly because “part of the fun at a ball game is to stuff yourself with junk food.”

Differentiate hunger, indicated by stomach contractions and an internally triggered need for food, from a response to totally external events that drive you to eat impulsively.

Drink lots of water, sparkling water, or other calorie-free drinks and chew gum!

Day 159

Behavior

To discourage impulsive eating, eat only after you set out a place mat, plate, drinking glass, coffee cup, flatware, and napkin at your "Designated Place," and then sit down.

Never eat standing up. No mindless eating standing in front of the refrigerator or by the stove. Sitting down signifies that you have made a conscious decision to eat. You are in control. You can then decide what and how much to eat.

Slow down and enjoy the food.

Day 160

Eat Slowly

To enjoy your delicious sandwich thoroughly, develop the new habit of taking small bites, putting the sandwich down on your plate after every single bite, and picking it up again only after you have chewed well and swallowed the previous morsel. Sip water between bites.

Keep up a lively conversation with dinner companions, lingering between morsels.

Day 161

At Work

If some of your colleagues are not supportive of your efforts to eat healthy meals and to improve your eating habits, be selective in the company that you keep for breaks and lunchtime.

If your co-workers are constantly tempting and testing you and sabotaging your good intentions, skip the group breaks and use the time to catch up on your personal correspondence, phone calls, paperwork, or reading.

Day 162

Eating Out

If you are dining by yourself, request that all appetizers, nuts, condiments, butter, and dressings be removed from your table. This will clearly convey your determination.

If you are dining with companions, have those items moved away from you to the far end of the table so they will be available for others.

If necessary, move them away yourself before you settle down.

Day 163

Dining Out

You are invited out. You have decided to skip the appetizer and to end your meal with a bowl of fresh berries, instead of a rich dessert. At the restaurant, you discover that you are entitled to a full-course dinner.

Stay firm with your decision. Do not indulge just because you are entitled or because it is already paid for. You always have the option to have some of it wrapped up to take home to have the next day.

The feeling of being in control and making a mature decision will be most gratifying.

Day 164

Dinner Parties

If you are going to a party late in the evening, make sure you do not arrive feeling ravenously hungry. A relatively comfortable stomach bolsters your determination, resolve, and discipline.

Before leaving home, have a generous helping of some vegetables, a piece of fruit, or a slice of whole-wheat bread, to blunt your hunger.

On a cold day, a cup of warm bullion or broth works wonders. Try it!

Day 165

Buffet Dinners

Look over the entire display of food on the table before you start helping yourself to whatever happens to be at the start of the buffet. Be selective. Choose small portions of your favorite dishes—the ones you would really enjoy.

Eat the foods you find truly delicious. If some of the items are not prepared to your satisfaction, do not eat them; leave them on your plate.

Mingle. You are not there for the food. You are there to visit with friends and meet people.

Day 166

Did You Know That?

A tossed salad with lettuce, tomato, cucumber, mushroom, red pepper, broccoli, shredded carrot, and two tablespoons grated cheese, with two tablespoons of low-calorie dressing comes to about 280 calories.

The same salad with added coleslaw, potato salad, macaroni salad, bacon bits, sunflower seeds, and croutons, with two tablespoons of regular dressing adds up to about 750 calories.

What is the right choice?

Day 167

Buying Food

Stay away from processed, prepared meals. They are usually high in saturated fat, total fat, salt, and total calories.

Read the labels on the ready-to-serve packages claiming to be low-fat, low-cholesterol, and low-calorie. Do not make any assumptions. Some brands of turkey hot dogs actually contain more fat than beef hot dogs.

Remember, for commercially prepared foods, "low-fat" does not necessarily mean "low-calorie."

Day 168

Grocery Shopping

Be an informed consumer of food. Read the package labels, especially for total fat and cholesterol content and calories.

The Food and Drug Administration requires all food manufacturers to use a standard Nutrition Facts label on their products. The new label is a great source of information about the nutritional content of the food. Read and compare with other products for total fat, saturated fat, cholesterol, sodium, total carbohydrates, sugar, fiber, protein, and calories per serving.

Day 169

A Sample of a Food Label from a Box of Cereal

Nutrition Facts
Serving Size 3/4 cup (31g)
Servings Per Container about 15

Amount Per Serving	Cereal	Cereal with 1/2 cup Skim Milk
Calories	130	170
Calories from Fat	25	25
	% Daily Value**	
Total Fat 2.5g*	**4%**	**4%**
Saturated Fat 0.5g	**3%**	**3%**
Cholesterol 0mg	**0%**	**0%**
Sodium 190mg	**8%**	**11%**
Potassium 60mg	**2%**	**7%**
Total Carbohydrate 24g	**8%**	**10%**
Dietary Fiber 1g	**4%**	**4%**
Sugars 7g		
Other Carbohydrate 16g		
Protein 3g		

Note: The average person eats 1 1/2 cups of cereal. With skim milk, that amounts to 340 calories. With 2 percent or whole milk, and a banana, it could add up to 500 calories.

Day 170

Storing Food

If your family must have those fat-laden, calorie-rich snacks available, store them in the kitchen or pantry cabinets, along with all other edibles. Do not display crackers, candy, nuts, finger foods, desserts, or other snacks in the living room, the family room, the study, or in the car.

Keep snacks away from areas where you spend long hours working on the computer, reading, writing, or watching television.

Day 171

Serving Food

Make a point of never nibbling or eating directly from a casserole, baking dish, pot, or frying pan.

Eating directly from the serving platter, whether in the kitchen or at the table, encourages overeating. It will be impossible for you to keep track of the amount you eat. You will not be able to stay within the calorie limit that you have set for yourself.

Use a plate at all times.

Day 172

Rewards

Evidence of a change in the right direction, however small, enhances your self-esteem, your happiness, and urges you on to stay committed.

Dwell on the positive. List the good eating habits you have adopted, the new physical activities you participate in, and the steady weight loss you have achieved.

Be proud of the new slimmer and trimmer person you have become.

Day 173

Reinforcement

Make new friends. Join new groups and get involved in their projects and activities. The more activity-oriented the group, the more desirable for your goals.

You can choose from so many possibilities such as hiking, mountain climbing, cycling, bowling, swimming, golf, canoeing, tennis, or team sports.

Live life to the fullest!

Day 174

Summary

Review and reinforce the simple, easy, and effective new habits that you have developed so far:

You will be enjoying your low-fat, high-fiber meals, sitting in the one designated spot at home and at work, table laid out, chewing small morsels slowly, sipping water, conversing with companions, concentrating on the joy of eating and savoring every bite.

Relish the wonderful feeling that you get from having accomplished something worthwhile.

Day 175

Review

Identify the diet tips that you have not been able to master yet. Pinpoint the new eating habits that you are having difficulty in practicing. List the modifications and changes you find challenging, and review them periodically for guidance.

Determine the tips that have been most helpful to you and refer to them for reinforcement.

Repetition is the key for developing new good habits.

Day 176

Goal

Write down a clear and concise statement of your goal. It will reinforce your motivation and commitment. Be specific. For example:

"I will weigh . . . lbs, wear size . . . clothes, walk . . . miles . . . times a week by . . . (date), and feel great by the occasion of . . ."

Picture yourself as the new trim and fit person you will be—visualize how you will look, dress, and act. See yourself impressing family, colleagues, and friends with your poise, energy, and self-confidence.

Day 177

Fat

Research indicates that the desire for fatty foods is an acquired or learned taste, a habit developed over many years of overindulgence. Therefore you can train yourself to gradually reduce the desire for fat-laden foods.

Habits can be changed by repetition and persistence. A generation ago everyone grew up drinking whole milk, and many found it difficult to switch to skim milk. Now most people actually prefer skim and consider whole milk too rich.

Day 178

Oil

Vegetable oils are, in general, healthier sources of fat because they usually contain polyunsaturated and monounsaturated fats.

Not all vegetable oils are better, though. Coconut oil, cocoa butter (the fat in chocolate), and palm oil contain highly saturated fats and should be avoided.

The popcorn sold at movie theaters is often drenched with butter-flavored coconut oil.

If you must have popcorn at the movie theater, ask for the one "without butter."

Day 179

Fat

All of the different cuts of meat contain substantial amounts of fat:

	Approximate Total Calories	Approximate Calories from Fat
4 oz. Sirloin Steak		
broiled, with fat	465	360
broiled, fat trimmed	235	170
4 oz. Hamburger		
broiled, regular	325	240
broiled, lean	250	120

Use less marbled and less fatty cuts of meat, and trim fat before and after cooking.

Day 180

Low-Fat Cooking Tips

Refrigerate chicken broth, stews and soups, and skim off the fat before using.

Season cooked vegetables or salads with herbs, spices, mustard, lemon juice, and balsamic vinegar instead of oily dressings.

Use low-fat, light or part-skim cheeses instead of cream cheese, ricotta cheese, or other whole-milk cheeses.

Day 181

Suggested Substitutions

Instead of	Use
Alcoholic beverages	Water, seltzer, club soda
Apple pie	Baked apple
Bread—white	Whole-wheat bread
Butter or animal fat	Vegetable oil, olive oil
Cheese—soft (Brie)	Hard Cheese (cheddar, Swiss)
Chocolate, candy bar	Dried fruit
Cream—heavy	Milk
Cream cheese	Low-fat cottage cheese
Creamy dressings	Lemon juice, vinegar, spices
Creamed soups	Consommé, bouillon, broth

Day 182

Preparing Food

If the food preferences and habits of your spouse and other family members are different from your new healthy eating habits, prepare your own meals and enjoy generous portions of a delicious light healthy fare.

Shop for your own needs and keep an ample supply of salad greens, fresh vegetables, fruit, potatoes, sweet potatoes, whole wheat pasta, beans, fat-free or low-fat dairy products, and salad dressings on hand. Be prepared to make your own special meals at short notice.

Day 183

Protein

Fish and shellfish are excellent sources of protein. Compared to other kinds of animal protein, most kinds of fish contain less fat, and moreover, the fat is low in saturated fat and high in polyunsaturated fat.

Method of preparation is crucial to keep it low-fat, low-calorie, and healthy.

4 oz., broiled	Approximate Calories
Cod, flounder, sole; fillet, no butter	90
Cod, flounder, sole; fillet, with butter	190
Shrimp; shelled, boiled	100
Shrimp; shelled, breaded, fried	250

Day 184

Protein

Animal protein sources usually cost considerably more than carbohydrate foods, such as potatoes, pasta, bread, rice, cereal, and beans.

Beans and legumes provide adequate protein, do not contain cholesterol, are much lower in fat content, and hence contain fewer calories gram for gram. Excessive animal protein is an expensive and wasteful way to get your energy.

Reduce animal protein and replace with beans and soybeans served with brown rice or whole-grain bread.

Day 185

Food You Should Eat

Beans: Rich in protein, iron, and fiber. Low in fat. Inexpensive.

Broccoli: Rich in vitamin C and fiber.

Cantaloupes, Oranges, Watermelon: Delicious and excellent sources of vitamin C.

Milk, fat-free or 1 percent fat: Excellent source of calcium, protein, and vitamins. Low in fat.

Oatmeal: Plain, old-fashioned, whole-grain oatmeal. Rich in vitamins and fiber.

Sweet Potatoes: One of the most nutritious vegetables. Loaded with vitamin C and fiber.

Whole grain bread: Rich in vitamins, minerals, and fiber.

Day 186

Lentil Soup (rich with protein)

2 14 oz. cans fat-free chicken broth
1 28 oz. can crushed tomatoes
1 cup whole lentils, washed
1/3 cup brown rice
1 onion, sliced
3 garlic cloves, minced
2 carrots, sliced thin
2 stalks celery, sliced thin
1 green/red pepper, sliced thin
1 pack frozen chopped spinach, thawed
juice of 1 lemon
pinch of cayenne
pinch of cumin
1 teaspoon salt
water

In a large pot, combine all ingredients. Bring to a boil, cover, and simmer for about forty minutes or until lentils are tender. Adjust spices to taste. If necessary, add water to get desired consistency.

(110-130 calories per cup. Negligible fat.)

Day 187

Priorities

If the owner's manual of your car stated "unleaded gasoline only," you wouldn't think of using anything else. You would fill up with unleaded gasoline only.

Your own health manual specifies "low-fat only." . . . And . . . you ignore it. You keep filling up on fatty, greasy food.

Set your priorities right. You are more important than your car. A car can always be replaced. There is only one of You. You are a special and unique person. Love yourself. Pamper yourself. Take good care of yourself.

Day 188

To Strengthen Your Resolve

Negative reinforcements could be put to good use too. You could work miracles with:

An unflattering photo displayed on your bathroom mirror or your refrigerator, or taped discreetly inside your closet door.

An embarrassing episode that was pivotal in your decision to lose the extra pounds.

A note of rejection, citing weight as a cause, that propelled you to the road to weight loss.

A statement of resolution you wrote.

Review these when the need arises.

Day 189

The Potato

It is what we do to the potato during food preparation that renders it "undesirable." A tablespoon of butter added, doubles the calories to 200. Served as potato chips, each ounce provides 160 calories. Just 5 ounces add up to 800 calories. A side order of one cup of French fries will add 450 calories.

Top the baked potato with two tablespoons of low-fat yogurt (20 calories) instead of butter or sour cream (200 calories).

Day 190

Sandwiches

For a delightful lunch, try pocket pita bread stuffed to overflowing with your favorite raw sliced vegetables—lettuce, cucumbers, tomatoes, cauliflower, broccoli, red or green peppers, onions, bean sprouts—with some balsamic vinaigrette or spicy mustard for flavor.

Thin slices of tofu, two slices of lean cold cuts, or some shredded cheese can be added to enhance protein content and flavoring.

Day 191

Sugar

Substituting honey, molasses, or fructose for ordinary sugar will defeat the purpose of reducing the craving and the rationalized need for sweets, because these are just as sweet and laden with empty calories too.

Avoid sugar-rich drinks. Regular sodas add up to an amazing number of calories each day. Replace sugar-loaded carbonated beverages with water, carbonated water, club soda, seltzer water, ice tea, or unsweetened fresh fruit juices.

Day 192

Healthy Dessert Suggestions:

Instead of ice cream and all its fat:

If you are fond of bananas, peel a delicious ripe one, slice it, arrange in a single layer on a small plate, and place in the freezer until just firm. Enjoy a delicious "Banana Ice."

Stock your freezer with packages of strawberries, raspberries, and blackberries, frozen whole, no sugar or syrup added. Thaw slightly at room temperature. "Berry Ice" will be ready to munch on and enjoy in minutes.

Day 193

Beverages

Beverage, 12 oz	Calories
Diet soda	3
Regular soda	120-150
Beer, regular	150
Wine	240
Vanilla shake	240
Chocolate shake	270

Sodas and shakes add too many empty calories devoid of nutritional value and are one of the major causes of childhood and adolescent obesity. Reserve them only for rare occasions.

Day 194

Fiber

The water-soluble fiber in foods such as beans, lentils, split peas, and oat bran, can effectively lower blood cholesterol levels and triglycerides. The daily soluble fiber requirement can be met by a cup of oat-bran cereal or a cup of cooked beans.

Natural unrefined complex carbohydrates are more effective than added bran. Insoluble fiber, such as wheat bran, has no effect on elevated cholesterol levels.

Day 195

Vitamins

Vitamins are essential natural ingredients that the body needs for healthy growth and normal function.

A diet of fresh vegetables, fresh fruit, citrus fruit, legumes, fortified milk, whole-grain bread, and protein from both animal and plant sources will provide the necessary vitamins.

The key to an adequate source of vitamins is variety in your diet. As a general rule, one multi-vitamin-and-mineral tablet and a vitamin C tablet a day are recommended. Always check with your physician regarding additional minerals—such as calcium—and antioxidants.

Day 196

Raw Vegetables

Whenever possible, eat your vegetables raw. Cabbage, carrots, celery, broccoli, cauliflower, zucchini, red and green bell peppers, and some mushrooms taste great without cooking, when served with a fat-free dip, fat-free dressing, or added to your various salads.

Wash these vegetables thoroughly. Rinse leafy ones in a heavy stream of water, and scrub those with hard surfaces, to remove pesticides.

Day 197

Energy

Sixty to 75 percent of calories burned each day are used for the energy required to run the body at rest, for growth, and for the replacement of used-up cells.

Another roughly 10 percent of the calories are used to digest and process the food eaten.

The remaining calories are used for physical activity, a significant amount of about 15 to 30 percent, over which we have the most control.

Day 198

Basal Metabolic Rate

When you are completely at rest, not involved in any physical activity, you will require energy for the basic functions of your body—such as breathing, keeping the heart pumping, maintaining body temperature, and digesting food. This energy requirement is known as the **Resting** or **Basal Metabolic Rate.** It varies for each individual based on genetic factors, gender, age and body size, and goes down gradually as you advance in age.

Since you also become physically less active as you progress in life, the total calorie needs of your body decrease steadily, and so does your need for food. Decrease the portions that you eat accordingly.

Day 199

Physical Activity

Physical activity raises the Metabolic Rate. You can reverse the gradual drop of your Basal Metabolic Rate by increasing your physical activity because regular exercise maximizes your metabolic calorie burn-off. **You burn calories not just while you are working out, but continuously for hours after you have stopped the exercise.**

For physical activity to be effective, consistency is crucial. Make exercise a regular part of your life.

Just get up and go! You owe it to yourself.

Day 200

Strength Training

Your Basal Metabolic Rate drops as the years go by because the proportion of fat relative to muscle in your body gradually increases as you get older. Fat tissue burns fewer calories compared to muscle tissue, which burns more energy.

A strength-training routine builds muscle. Exercising with weights replaces the fat with muscle, which revs up your metabolism, substantially increasing the number of calories you burn each day.

Weight training is also the most effective way to increase bone density. Not only will you lose fat and gain muscle, you will also reduce your risk of osteoporosis.

Work out with weights. It's good for you!

Day 201

Calories

If you have not yet kept records of food intake and physical activity, it is important that you do so for your own benefit.

Jot down the approximate total calorie content of the food and drinks consumed each day for a "typical" week, then calculate your daily average. If this number of calories resulted in pounds of fat creeping up on you quietly but steadily over the years, you are eating far too much and exercising too little.

Persistence is the key to your success. Be persistent and you will reach your goal.

Day 202

Walking

If frequent leisurely walking is already part of your established routine, increase the length and frequency of your walks, and focus on walking at a faster pace, until you get to walk briskly for thirty minutes, three times a week.

If you are looking for new challenges, you can further improve your workout by walking uphill, by swinging your arms fully or even adding some wrist or ankle weights.

You will feel so good that you will eventually want to exercise rather than have to exercise. You will enjoy the journey to fitness as much as reaching the destination itself.

Day 203

Physical Activity

In case of inclement weather:

—Follow exercise and fitness programs offered daily on some television stations.
—Use an exercise routine on video and work out with the experts.
—Use a stationary bicycle and exercise at home.
—Use a treadmill and work out indoors.
—Join a health club.

Almost any consistent activity will do, provided you follow it regularly and build it up to a good pace.

Get involved in a variety of activities to make it more interesting.

Day 204

Physical Activity

Some people are overweight, not because they eat too much, but because they exercise too little.

Physical activity is essential, but be patient. Start at a slow pace and progress gradually. Be aware of your body's physical warning signs while you exercise. Never push yourself to the point of being short of breath. Stop at the first hint of fatigue, pain, or discomfort, especially if you have just started exercising after a long period of sedentary living. Be patient and persist.

Day 205

Bicycling

You can get a good workout bicycling outdoors or on an indoor stationary bicycle. Compared to walking, and especially jogging, bicycling is less stressful on the ankles, feet, and knees unless you cycle uphill. With the indoor bike, you can simulate easier or harder paths.

Health clubs offer a large variety of exercise machines simulating walking, jogging, cross-country skiing, stair climbing, weight training, and many others. Choose a variety of workouts that you find enjoyable, to insure persistence and long-term benefits.

Day 206

Hunger

It is counterproductive to eat in anticipation of feeling hungry. If not hungry, do not eat to avoid getting hungry later on. Wait until you actually feel the need for nourishment.

Do not snack with the excuse of backup energy before you exercise.

Identify the situations in which you eat even though you are not hungry; and avoid repeating the old habits, one habit at a time. **Eat only when hungry.**

Day 207

Behavior

If you think you are turning to food for a break from routine work, or because of procrastination facing an unpleasant task, admit to yourself that food cannot and does not alleviate emotional stress or boredom. On the contrary, it aggravates the initial stress, often adding feelings of guilt.

Before you snack ask yourself: "Why do I feel like eating?" If you are not hungry, instead of eating, drink a glass of water, make a phone call, or run an errand.

Day 208

Emotions

If you are snacking because of	You are expecting food to give you
Boredom	Recreation
Frustration	Peace
Anger, upset	Serenity
Anxiety	Security
Loneliness	Companionship
Sadness	Happiness

You are eating to avoid facing personal conflicts and to compensate for the emotional dilemma with temporary gratification.

Admit you are turning to food merely as a substitute and for distraction from the real issue; pinpoint your particular emotional need and work on solving that problem.

Day 209

Behavior Pattern Records

List the behavior patterns that contribute to overeating. What activities or places make you reach for a snack automatically? Do you go to the refrigerator as soon as you return home? Do you reach for a snack as soon as you turn the television on?

Just being aware of these patterns marks the beginning of gradually decreasing and eventually eliminating wrong habits altogether.

Day 210

At Work

If you cannot bring your own lunch, and at lunch break you find that you lose all resolve when you are exposed to the aroma and array of dishes in the cafeteria, ask a friend to buy a clearly specified low-calorie meal for you.

Avoid the display of tempting choices altogether; go directly to the sitting area and wait there for your supportive friend.

Day 211

Eating Out

Be the first one at the table to order your food, so as not to be influenced by the choices of the others. Order a la carte, not the full-course dinner. You might order:

—An entree only, without the appetizer, soup, or salad. Fresh fruit for dessert.
—An appetizer and a large salad for an entree. A scoop of sorbet for dessert.
—In addition to your appetizer, order another appetizer instead of an entrée. A cup of coffee.

Place your entire order at once and do not change your mind later on.

Day 212

Clearing Plates

You are under no obligation to eat all that is on your plate. You do not have to "clear your plate". You decide how much you should eat; no one else has the authority to make that decision for you.

When you determine you have had all you want to eat, put your napkin down with determination to indicate that you have finished eating. Don't nibble at leftover food.

Day 213

Learn to Be More Assertive

Celebrate special occasions with friends who share your passion for healthy eating and respect your choices.

Socialize with friends who will support you and encourage you to stay firm in your commitment to an active lifestyle. Hang out with those who enjoy outdoor adventures and participate in projects that involve activity.

Let people know how you feel about food, eating, and participating in projects that involve activity. Express your opinion clearly and remain steadfast in your determination.

Day 214

Dinner Parties

Plan ahead. Reserve calories for this special occasion by having a small breakfast and a light lunch. Allocate the balance to the fancy meal that evening. You can even plan to eat less the day before or the day after, to feel truly in control.

Have a firm plan ahead of time as to the healthy items you will select and the categories of foods you will avoid, such as the fried greasy hors d'oeuvres being passed around and the rich creamy desserts.

Day 215

On Vacations

Plan ahead. Stay away from the ocean liners, where the focus is on continuous eating for the entire duration.

When planning vacations, make it clear to your spouse, partner, family, or friends, long before arrangements are made, that you are not interested in the cruises that are geared for senseless overeating.

Suggest vacation spots where walking trails, nature walks, tennis courts, and golf courses are available, and meals are not included in the prepaid package deal.

Day 216

The Food Label

Read it carefully. A sample on a can of soup:

Nutrition Facts	
Serving size	1cup
Servings per container	about 2 1/2
Amount per Serving	
Calories	140
Calories from Fat	20
Total Fat	2 g
Saturated Fat	0 g
Cholesterol	5 mg
Sodium	750 mg
Total Carbohydrate	22 g
Dietary Fiber	7 g
Sugar	2 g
Protein	9 g

Most people eat the entire can of soup. That would amount to 350 calories.

Day 217

Suggested Substititions

Instead of	Use
Apple juice, orange juice	Apples, oranges
Desserts	Fresh fruit
Eggs, scrambled	Poached eggs
French fries	Baked potatoes
Fruit, canned in syrup	Fruit, canned in juice
Frying, batter frying	Steaming, boiling, broiling, grilling
Gravy	Bouillon, broth
Ice Cream	Frozen fresh fruit
Mayonnaise	Olive oil, yogurt

Day 218

Serving Food

Help yourself to the amount of food that you have decided to eat. Keep the pot, casserole, or serving platter away from the table.

Sip your water and eat your portion slowly, enjoying every morsel. If you still feel hungry**, and decide to have some more, go back into the kitchen and help yourself again.**

The additional eating should be a conscious and deliberate decision, not an automatic, mindless action.

Day 219

Storing Leftovers

If you hosted a dinner party or reception, prepare hostess packages with the excess appetizers and desserts for your guests to take home.

Send packages to family members or friends who could not make the party.

Store leftovers in the freezer. Frozen food will not present as ready a temptation at a weak moment.

In Summary:

—Count every calorie, solid and liquid.
—Limit calorie intake to less than calorie expenditure.
—Decrease the amount of total fat intake.
—Replace most animal fat with vegetable oils.
—Replace animal protein with plant protein.
—Decrease red meat, replace with fish, chicken, and turkey.
—Eat more of complex carbohydrates, whole-grain breads, and legumes.
—Increase fresh vegetables, seeds, roots, bulbs, and fruit.

Keep up with your regular physical activity.

Recognize every dietary adjustment you make as a personal triumph.

Day 221

Minestrone

- 2 cans fat-free chicken broth
- 1 28-oz can crushed tomatoes
- 1 potato
- 2 carrots
- 1 celery stalk
- 1 onion
- 1/2 red pepper
- 2 cloves garlic
- 1/2 cup pasta
- 1 cup water
- 2 tbsp olive oil
- 1 can white beans
- 1 can kidney beans
- 1 can chick peas
- 1 can peas
- juice of 1 lemon
- 1/2 tsp salt
- 1/4 tsp thyme
- 1/4 tsp oregano
- pinch of cayenne

In a large pot, start heating the chicken broth and tomatoes. Chop and add potatoes, carrots, celery, onion, pepper, and garlic. Bring to a boil. Add pasta and simmer for fifteen minutes. Add drained beans, peas, and spices. Simmer five more minutes. Adjust seasonings. Add more water if desired. Serve hot.

(90-110 calories per cup. Minimal fat.)

Note: You can vary the amounts of the vegetables as desired.

Day 222

Reflections

Remember that **setbacks are positive learning experiences;** they are not indications of failure.

Learn from each setback. Figure out what happened, why it happened, and under what circumstances you have to be especially determined and steadfast.

Gain insight from the experience and get back on track. Persist and you will definitely achieve your goal.

Give yourself credit for what you have achieved so far. Be proud of your accomplishment.

Day 223

Goal

Remember the turtle?

Set a slow-paced goal. Remember that you gained the extra pounds gradually, slowly, and steadily in small increments, over many years.

Your body will eliminate the unwanted pounds in exactly the same way as they crept up on you—slowly, gradually, and in small increments, over the many months and years ahead, depending on your specific case.

Be determined, persistent, and patient.

Day 224

Rewards

As an added incentive, set aside and save the money that you would have wasted on potato chips, peanuts, candy bars, doughnuts, steaks, and the like.

With the accumulated savings, treat yourself occasionally with the luxury of a manicure, a pedicure, a relaxing facial, or an invigorating body massage.

Pamper yourself. Appreciate yourself. When you have already given praise to yourself, you do not need to hear it from others.

Day 225

Dairy Products

Milk is a great source of nutrition. It is important to remember that all the various choices offered provide the same nutrients, the only difference being the fat content. The fat you do not need.

	Percent Fat by weight	Approximate Calories per cup
Whole Milk	3.5	160
Low-fat milk	2	120–140
Low-fat milk	1	110–115
Skim	0.1	80–90

Replace whole milk with low-fat milk, and eventually skim milk, to cut down on fat and calories, but still enjoy the wholesome nutrients, protein and calcium in milk.

Day 226

Low-fat Food Preparation Tips

Use skim or low-fat milk instead of whole milk. Use non-fat or low-fat yogurt instead of whole-milk yogurt.

Use plain yogurt instead of sour cream, especially for salad dressings, dips, toppings, and baked potatoes.

Replace ice cream with sherbet, ice milk, frozen yogurt, or sorbet for desserts.

Day 227

Fat

Rest assured that low-fat cooking does not mean tasteless or boring food. On the contrary, you will find that your meals will taste richer with variety, because you will taste the individual and distinctive flavors of the items rather than the butter itself.

You will discover a new range of flavors and develop a new appreciation for simple, natural nourishment. The healthy food choices will become desirable and enjoyable.

Day 228

Oil

Health-conscious individuals often turn to "non-dairy creamers" for their coffee, in their effort to eliminate cream and milk fat.

Beware of most commercial "non-dairy creamers." They are typically made with coconut oil, which is a very highly saturated vegetable oil.

Always read the list of ingredients—total fat, saturated fat—before buying these products. As a possible alternative, check the new products that claim to be "non-fat coffee creamers."

Day 229

Reflections

Take responsibility for your own actions; it is crucial for losing weight and successfully keeping it off.

You have to want to lose the weight for yourself. You must believe deeply that you deserve to become the trim and lively person that you can be. You must be convinced that you can definitely achieve it.

You are important. You deserve better than the treatment you have given yourself so far. Pamper yourself.

Compliment yourself. Positive thoughts create a self-fulfilling prophecy.

Day 230

Cholesterol

Animal fat consists mostly of saturated fat, which metabolizes and results in an increase in blood cholesterol levels. Limiting animal fat intake not only reduces total calorie intake but also helps lower blood cholesterol levels. It is therefore desirable, not only from the point of view of weight reduction, but also for cardiovascular health and overall healthy living.

To limit saturated fat intake, stay away from lard, pork, bacon, most red meats, butter, creamy cheeses, and milk fat. Eat smaller portions of these items and make up the difference with legumes, grains, and vegetables.

Day 231

Oil

"Partially hydrogenated vegetable oils" are oils treated by the hydrogenation process, which hardens the liquid oils, making them easier to spread. Margarine is an example. However, this chemical process changes the beneficial polyunsaturated fats of plant origin into undesirable "trans" fats.

These hydrogenated oils do not fall in the category of desirable oils of plant origin any more. They should be treated as saturated fats, which raise cholesterol levels, promote heart disease, and must be avoided. Study the labels on margarine packages.

Day 232

Behavior

Before you eat high-calorie treats, ask yourself, "Is the temporary pleasure of eating this, worth the calories?" If you decide that it is, then enjoy every morsel. If it is not, then substitute.

You can never go wrong by substituting fresh raw vegetables and fruit for calorie-laden snacks and desserts. When in doubt, reach for one of nature's fresh gifts. Have an apple, a pear, or an orange for a snack, instead of the half-cup of peanuts that will cost you 800 calories. You could eat an entire satisfying meal with those calories.

Day 233

Soy Products

Most supermarkets now carry “veggie burgers,” “garden vegetable patties,” and “meatless burgers, grillers, and franks.” Made from soybeans, vegetables, herbs and spices, these products can be good sources of vegetable protein. Try them for taste.

Read the “Nutrition Facts” very carefully since some of these products can be high in fat content.

Textured Vegetable Protein (TVP), a soy protein concentrate, in the form of flakes or granules, can be added to soups and salads or used in recipes as a substitute for ground beef.

Day 234

Cheese

Cheese is a good source of protein. However, most varieties are also high in fat content and cholesterol. Some creamy varieties have higher fat and cholesterol content than not only fish and poultry, but even red meat!

Scan labels carefully and select wisely from the wider variety available, because their fat content varies enormously. Select the "part-skim" and harder varieties.

Day 235

Potato Toppings

You might want to experiment with the many "low-fat" and "fat-free" products now crowding the supermarket shelves. Your choices include fat-free sour cream, butter-flavored flakes and sprays, fat-free or low-fat cottage cheese, and other products as toppings for baked potatoes. It is a matter of personal taste and preference. Onions, garlic, and a mix of your favorite vegetables sautéed in their own juices make yummy toppings.

You will also find fat-free mayonnaise for potato salad.

Day 236

Bread

The calorie content of bread is about 60 to 80 per slice. There are now many low-calorie whole-grain breads available with only 40 to 60 calories per slice. Compare:

Food Choices	Calories	Equivalent Number of Slices of Bread	
		Regular	Low-Cal
Cheese, 2 oz	200	2-3	4-5
Cold Cuts, 2 oz	180	2-3	3-4
Potato chips, 2 oz	320	4-5	6-7

Two ounces of potato chips, adding 320 calories, will neither give you the bulk and fiber, nor satisfy your hunger and fill you up, the way the two slices of bread in your sandwich will, for half the calories.

Day 237

Sugar

Sugar does provide readily available and easily absorbed calories that might give a false sense of satisfaction and a quick surge of energy. But it also stimulates the secretion of insulin. Chronic high levels of insulin stimulate hunger, thus causing a further desire for food.

Insulin also slows down the burning of body fat and instead promotes the synthesis and deposit of fat.

Stay away from the sweetened "regular" soft drinks, shakes, and desserts, like the 670-calorie Cinnabon.

Day 238

Healthy Snack and Dessert Suggestions

For a quick healthy snack to replace candy bars, doughnuts, and rich pastries laden with fat and calories, have

—Sweet raisins
—Delicious dried apricots
—Tasty pitted prunes
—Yummy whole pitted dates
—Plain frozen berries
—Frozen banana slices

Day 239

Calories

Food intake increases the body's metabolic rate. Each time you eat a meal, your body revs up in order to digest the food and starts to burn calories at a slightly higher rate. Hence by spreading your food intake over several small meals during the day, you will burn calories more efficiently.

Do not skip breakfast and lunch so you will not end up eating a huge dinner in the evening. Have three regular meals a day.

Day 240

Food Fiber

The increased bulk and roughage contributed by meals with high fiber content speed up the passage of food though the alimentary tract. Fiber acts as a natural laxative in the intestine, eliminating constipation and lowering the risk of cancer of the bowel and other complications.

Whenever possible, choose vegetables, whole grain products, legumes, and fruit over processed food.

Day 241

Antioxidants

Vitamins A, C, and E are some of the antioxidants that prevent certain oxidizing chemical reactions that produce the so-called free radicals that can be harmful to the body.

The best sources for these vitamins are yellow and orange vegetables and citrus fruits. Eat generous helpings of these vegetables and fruits daily.

If you are not following a diet high in complex carbohydrates and whole grains, it would be wise to take one combination antioxidant tablet a day. Always check with your physician.

Day 242

Salt

Salt, in small quantities, is essential for the proper functioning of our body physiology. But excessive salt can aggravate high blood pressure and water retention, leading to cardiac problems. Sodium is the culprit.

High salt content is typical of the current American diet. **Stop the habit of automatically adding salt to your food before even tasting it. Gradually decrease the amount of the salt you add at the table. Eventually, aim at putting away the salt shaker entirely.**

Day 243

Summary

Let vegetables, fruit, whole grains, and legumes dominate your diet.

Eat fish, poultry, lean meats, nuts, seeds, olive oil, lowfat milk, cheese, and yogurt in moderation.

Consume whole milk, butter, creamy cheeses, eggs, and fatty meats in limited amounts.

Keep sweets, desserts, fat, and alcoholic beverages to an absolute minimum.

Day 244

The USDA Food Guide Pyramid

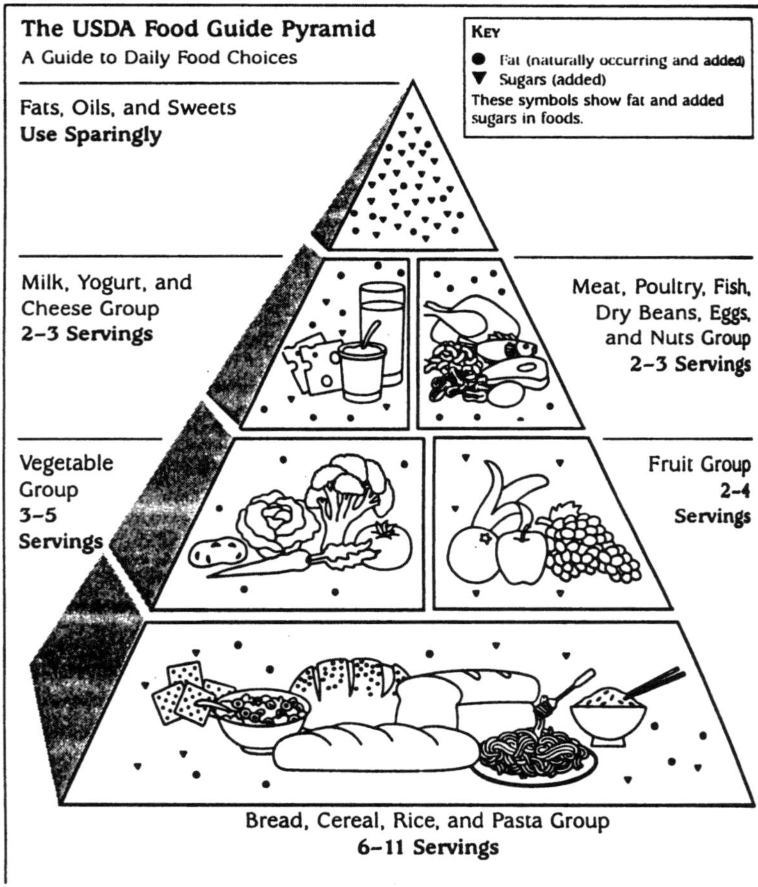

Day 245

The Food Pyramid

The United States Department of Agriculture pyramid has four tiers:

On the first and second tiers, we find grain products, vegetables, and fruits, foods that can be used freely as the foundation of a meal.

On the third tier—on one side dairy products and on the other side meats, poultry, fish, dry beans, eggs, and nuts, foods that should be used in smaller amounts and less frequently.

The top tier has fats, oils, and sweets—foods to be used sparingly.

Day 246

Keep Records

Clinical studies have shown that of all the people on diets, including diabetics, those who are successful keep dietary, weight, and activity records regularly. They are therefore well aware of their eating habits and are in a position to have control over what they eat.

List everything that you eat and record your daily physical activity. Weigh yourself once a week. These are your personal and confidential records and must be accurate in order to be useful and constructive.

Make every day count!

Day 247

Calories

There are charts that list recommended daily calorie intake based on gender, height, and build of an individual. But the basal metabolic rate and physiologic requirements vary so widely from person to person that it is better to figure out the specific amount for yourself.

If you have been keeping records as recommended earlier in this program, you can get a pretty good idea of your average daily total consumption calories.

Make the necessary changes and reduce the total amount to achieve your desired goal.

Day 248

Calories

Do not follow a restricted diet dictated by someone else.

Develop your own personalized diet by selecting the healthier, low-fat, low-calorie items from among the foods you like and enjoy eating.

Eat a wide variety of foods, including generous servings of the vegetables, legumes, and fruit that you relish. You will **develop good, lifelong eating habits for slow and steady weight loss and weight maintenance.**

You have the power to change your life. Use that power.

Day 249

Physical Activity

Ideally every intensive physical activity routine should consist of four phases:

—**Warm-up:** A few minutes of gentle movement and activity to warm up the muscles, followed by
—**Stretching,** to avoid tearing or damage to the muscles. Then,
—**The workout itself,** followed by
—**Cool-down:** A gradual slowing down of the same activity, in contrast to stopping suddenly.

Relax! Breathe deeply!

Exercise will satisfy your body and soul, and will become a cherished highlight of your life.

Day 250

Warm-Up

Warm-up exercises increase the blood supply to the heart and the muscles involved in that particular activity, thereby increasing the oxygen supply for energy, and making the muscles more pliable and more resistant to injury.

To warm-up, exercise at a relaxed pace the same muscles that you will be using for your workout such as walking slowly for a brisk walk or jogging for strenuous running.

Day 251

Stretching

Stretching will start the muscles working slowly and gradually, increase muscle flexibility, and reduce the possibility of injury.

After warm-up slowly stretch the muscles that you will be using most for the specific workout, such as calf and leg muscles for walking, jogging, or running or arm and leg muscles for swimming.

Day 252

Cooling Down

After completing your workout, continue the same activity at a slower pace to allow your body to cool down gradually and to get back to normal heartbeat and blood circulation. After running briskly, slow down to a jog, then walk, and gradually slow down to a stop.

The few minutes of slow exercise at the end of your workout gives your body a chance to ease back to its relaxed state.

Day 253

Hunger

Hunger is a normal and natural feeling. It is essential for life and survival. It is the mechanism through which your body indicates its normal need for nourishment.

If you don't feel hungry at your regular mealtime, do not eat your meal mechanically. Wait until you actually feel hungry, then relish every bite you take.

Day 254

Liquid Fillers

You can begin at least one meal a day with a bowl of low-fat or non-fat soup. Most bouillon and vegetable soups are nutritious, contain little fat, and are filling. Thus they will help reduce your appetite. As a result you will eat less.

Stay away from cream-based soups completely. Ideally, prepare your own vegetable soup in bulk, without any fat, and enjoy it routinely as your first course at mealtime.

Day 255

Behavior

It is not easy to forget old habits that you have practiced over the years. Eliminating an established behavior pattern and replacing it with another, always elicits resistance at first. However, it is also true that just as the old habits were developed with practice and repetition, **new and desirable ones can now replace them through practice, repetition, and reinforcement.**

Eat only in your designated place to make sure it will be the only one associated with eating.

Day 256

Eating Out

The Cocktail Hour

Alcohol is a concentrated source of calories with little nutritional value. Do not waste precious calories on alcohol when you can use those calories for healthy, filling, satisfying and nutritious food instead.

You can socialize just as elegantly sipping a glass of club soda with a twist of lime, a diet soft drink, iced tea, or any other low-calorie drink. Save the calories for your main course.

If you must have hard liquor, plan for it, and pass up dessert.

Day 257

Eating Out

The Appetizer.

If you are dining by yourself, just the entrée itself will satisfy your hunger, your nutritional needs, and your caloric limit. Skip the appetizer and soup.

If your companions are having appetizers, order a salad without any dressing on it. Ask for fresh lemon, vinegar, mustard, and olive oil; or ask for "the dressing on the side." Use the lemon, vinegar, and mustard generously and, if you must, only one tablespoon of the oil. Or use just one tablespoon of the dressing.

The salad will help curb your appetite with minimal calorie intake.

Day 258

Eating Out

The Main Course.

Order poultry or fish for your entrée rather than pork ribs or beefsteak, and **request that it be either baked, broiled, or grilled without any butter or oil. Discard any fat and skin.**

Order the **baked potato** instead of French fries or mashed potatoes. Skip the sour cream, the gravy, and the butter. Use spices, herbs, mustard, or sautéed vegetables instead.

Day 259

Eating Out

Dessert.

Learn to think of coffee as the end of a meal. If you must have something sweet, you can:

—Order a bowl of luscious berries.
—Choose a low-calorie item like "fruit in gelatin"
—Have one scoop of frozen yogurt.
—Share a "light" dessert with a friend.
—**Train yourself to stop after three morsels of the dessert and push the plate away resolutely.**

Day 260

On Vacation

Plan ahead: Let the people in your party know that you definitely plan to follow your healthy eating habits. Let them know that **being on vacation does not mean taking a vacation from sensible eating.** Ask them to respect your decision and not try to entice you with their choices or to rationalize with you about "being on vacation" and "enjoying yourself with total abandon."

Stick with your decision. Your friends will be impressed with your determination and discipline. **You will return home feeling wonderful about yourself.**

Day 261

Goal

Set a long-term goal. The new dietary adaptations will feel natural and comfortable to you only when practiced over a reasonably long period of time. Think of losing the weight over months and years. You want these new habits to become second nature to you so that you will adhere to them for the rest of your healthy and trim life, never reverting to the old wrong habits.

Experience each stage of development of the new exciting individual emerging.

You've made it work. Good for you!

Day 262

Occasional Lapses

Be comfortable with the idea of an occasional deviation from an idealized hard and fast plan of sensible eating and regular exercise. Such a lapse is not evidence of weakness or failure.

When you slip, take it in stride, assess the situation, and take immediate control to make sure things do not get out of hand. Instead of blaming yourself or faulting others, get back on track to prevent a lapse from becoming a relapse.

Delight in what you have accomplished so far. Celebrate your success.

Day 263

Cholesterol

Food package labels declaring “Contains No Cholesterol” are misleading. Read the listing of the ingredients. If the prepared food contains saturated fat, the latter will metabolize and still result in an increase of blood cholesterol levels.

Check the “Nutrition Facts” labels on the packages of prepared foods for fat content and refrain from using those containing high levels of fat, especially saturated fat.

Day 264

Cholesterol

The fat in animal flesh contains relatively high ratios of saturated fat, which will metabolize and increase the amount of already existing cholesterol. Almost all seafood, however, contains relatively less cholesterol and saturated fat and a higher percentage of unsaturated fat. In addition, it provides fish oils, which are beneficial.

Gradually replace pork and red meat with fish, and develop a taste for seafood rich in variety and flavors.

Day 265

Cheese

Currently supermarkets carry many “skim” or “reduced calorie” varieties—“low-fat” or “fat-free” cottage cheese, “light” or “fat-free” cream cheese or “part-skim” mozzarella. Whenever possible, without compromising flavor, substitute the lighter, low-fat varieties, and use them sparingly as condiments, shredded or thinly sliced rather than in chunks.

Day 266

Sugar

Taste is a matter of habit, and taste preferences can and do change over time.

Use less sugar in your coffee, tea, iced tea, lemonade, and other drinks. Reduce the amount of sugar that your recipes call for. After a while, your old favorites will taste too sweet to your refined taste buds. You will prefer the healthier, more nutritious choices that are also lower in calories.

Ideally, desserts should consist of fresh fruit, fruit gelatin, dried fruit, or fruit compotes cooked in their own juices, eliminating any sugar, butter, or whipped cream.

Day 267

The Food Pyramid

The USDA four-tier food pyramid previously shown has some shortcomings.

Beans, other legumes, and nuts are all clustered together on the third tier, along with meats, poultry, and fish, although these foods have quite different types and amounts of fat.

No distinction is made between low-fat or non-fat desirable milk products and whole milk products high in saturated fat that should be used only in moderation.

No differentiation is made between “good” oils, such as olive oil or other vegetable oils, and butter or animal fats that should be used only occasionally and in very small quantities.

Day 268

The Superpyramid

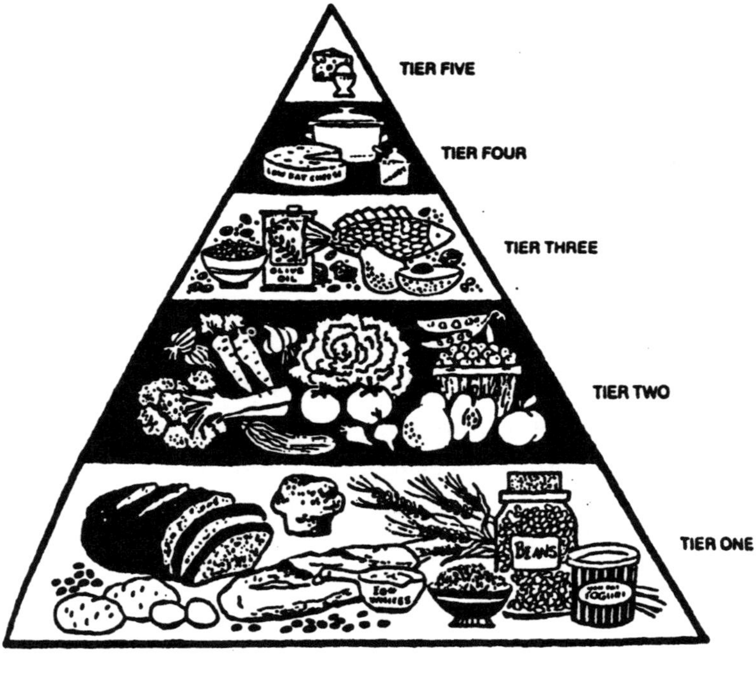

(From Spiller, Gene, Ph.D., *The Superpyramid Eating Program*. New York: Random House, 1993. Reprinted with permisison of the Sphera Foundation and Gene Spiller.)

Day 269

The Superpyramid

The advantages of the five-tier Superpyramid: It

—Makes a distinction between dairy products based on their fat content, placing them on three different tiers.
—Places beans, non-fat or low-fat milk products, and egg whites on the first tier, among grains and cereals, foods that can be eaten freely as important sources of protein and energy.
—Separates fish from other animal flesh, such as meat and poultry.

Day 270

The Superpyramid

The First Tier includes **whole-grain breads, whole-grain pasta, whole-grain cereals, brown rice, beans, other legumes, potatoes, corn, egg whites, and non-fat or low-fat yogurt and milk products.**

These are the basic foods for life, the foundation of your meals. In their unrefined form, these provide ample complex carbohydrates, protein, vegetable fat, fiber, vitamins, minerals, iron, and calcium. These foods can be eaten freely to meet your daily energy requirements.

Day 271

The Superpyramid

The Second Tier includes **vegetables and fruit —preferably eaten fresh and raw**—that supply complex carbohydrates, vitamins, minerals, and lots of fiber. These foods supplement the nutrients of the foods found on the First Tier and are just as vital to good health.

Fortunately, the variety of available vegetables and fruit is exciting and endless. Enjoy these vegetables in generous amounts.

Keep up the good work!

Day 272

The Superpyramid

The Third Tier contains **nuts, olives, avocados, and seeds.** These foods should be used in moderation to supplement the nutrients supplied by the foods on the first two tiers.

These plant foods supply precious oils, such as olive oil, sunflower oil, and sesame seed oil, to replace the harmful animal fats that you will be eliminating from your diet.

The Third Tier also includes fish as a healthy source of protein and fish oils.

Day 273

The Superpyramid

The Fourth Tier includes:

—Low-fat cheeses and other low-fat dairy products that supply excellent protein and calcium.
—Natural sweeteners, such as honey, maple syrup, molasses, and dark brown sugar, to add flavoring in small quantities.
—Low-fat meat and skinless poultry to be used as condiments in small amounts.

Day 274

The Superpyramid

The Fifth Tier includes:

—Whole eggs to be used in limited amounts only, especially by those who have high blood cholesterol levels. One whole egg, two egg whites, and lots of vegetables make a delicious omelet.
—Medium-fat cheeses and other medium-fat milk products used in small amounts add excellent flavor to enhance a dish without adding too many calories or too much saturated fat.

Day 275

Calories

Crash diets are neither healthy nor effective. They restrict the dieter to a few specific foods, eliminate entire nutrients completely, are nutritionally deficient, and can cause serious health problems. In addition, crash diets make the dieter feel deprived, craving for the wrong kinds of food, eager to end the ordeal, and revert to old habits.

Prepare foods that you enjoy eating. Reduce the amount of fat that the recipes call for, use less animal protein, more legumes and vegetables. Eat smaller portions.

Day 276

Keep Track of Calories

People who overeat are often unaware of how much or how often they eat. They nibble while baking, reading, working, or watching television, not because of hunger, but simply out of habit.

You realize by now that you are doing better at weight control when you keep track of your food intake. If you are getting lazy and slacking off, renew your commitment and keep your journal so you can measure your progress and identify the hurdles you encounter.

Just do it!

Day 277

Reflections

Define success as more than just reaching the weight that you have set as a goal.

Focus on **permanent positive lifestyle change** and not only weight loss.

Aim at eating healthy, at increasing physical activity, and feeling good about yourself for the rest of your life. You deserve the best.

You will lead a wholesome healthy life with many reasons to celebrate your unique personal achievement.

Day 278

Swimming

If you are a good swimmer and can do laps at a steady consistent rate, swimming would work wonders for you.

Swimming effectively exercises all major muscle groups at low risk of injury. It is ideal for those who are overweight, or have joint problems or arthritis, because the buoyancy of the water makes the body lighter and movement easier.

Aquatic exercise classes would work wonders if you enjoy group activities.

Day 279

Physical Activity

Exercise is also a natural appetite suppressant. When you work out regularly, you tend to eat less because you feel less hungry.

In fact, a good time to exercise is just before dinner. You will feel less ravenous and will be satiated with smaller portions.

Personalize your workout to fit your time and schedule. Be selfish. Do it for yourself.

Day 280

Behavior

If at a specific time of day you get a craving for something sweet, or you have a strong urge for a rich snack, plan to run your errands at around that time; get out of the house and away from food.

Better still, plan to take your daily walk at this specific time or day. You will not only avoid eating the extra calories, but you will burn some of your reserves instead. The craving will have passed by the time you get back.

Day 281

Keep Records

Self-monitoring develops the skills and attitude that are the foundation of self-change. It enables you to see in black and white your food preferences, eating habits, serving sizes, and your level of activity. In addition to eliminating self-deception, it helps you take responsibility for your actions and encourages you to take charge, to make an objective assessment, and implement the necessary changes, adjustments, and improvements.

Those who have been successful in losing weight have achieved it on their own.

More power to you.

Day 282

The Traditional Healthy Mediterranean Diet Pyramid

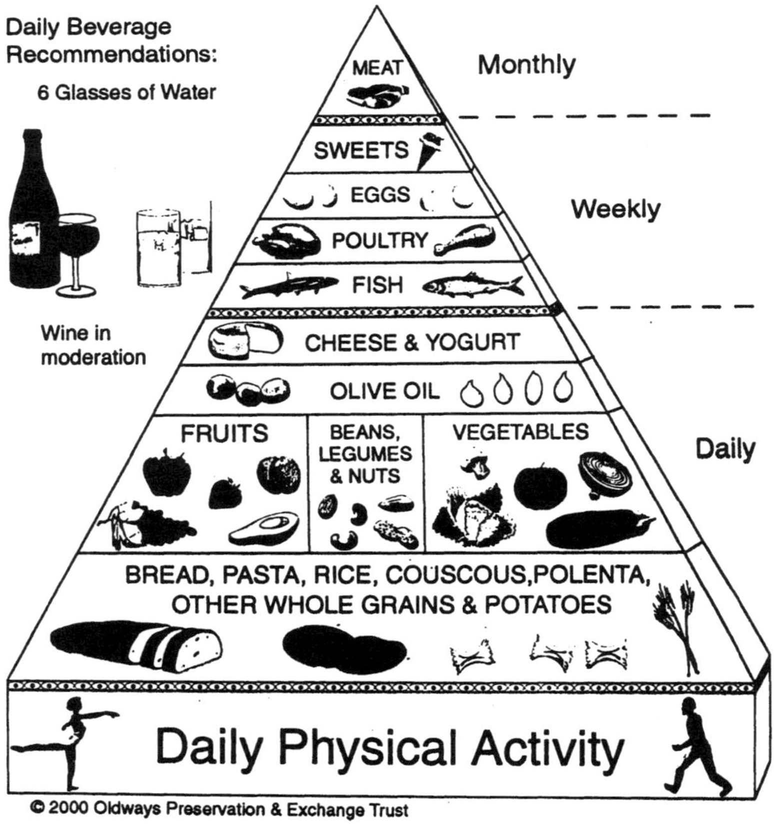

Day 283

The Mediterranean Diet Pyramid

Advantages

—An abundance of food from plant sources, including fruits and vegetables, potatoes, breads and grains, beans, nuts, and seeds.
—Emphasis on a variety of minimally processed and seasonally fresh foods.
—Olive oil as the principal fat, replacing other fats and oils such as butter and margarine.
—Total fat ranging from less than 25 to over 35 percent of energy, with saturated fat no more than 7 to 8 percent of calories.
—Daily consumption of low to moderate amounts of cheese and yogurt.
—Weekly consumption of low to moderate amounts of fish and poultry; zero to four eggs per week (including those used in cooking and baking).
—Fresh fruit as the typical daily dessert; sweets with sugar and saturated fat consumed not more than a few times per week.
—Red meat a few times per month.
—Regular physical activity promoting a healthy weight, fitness, and well-being.
—Moderate consumption of wine, normally with meals.

Day 284

The Cocktail "Hour"

Arrive fashionably late—that's what celebrities do. To minimize the chance for temptation, do not spend much time lingering around the bar.

Ideally, avoid all alcoholic drinks. Enjoy a tall glass of club soda, sparkling water, or seltzer water with a twist of lime, or sip your favorite diet soft drink. Save the calories for your dinner.

If you absolutely must have a cocktail, or a glass of wine, limit it to one and sip it s-l-o-w-l-y.

Day 285

Eating Out

Take advantage of the fact that most restaurants now offer “low-calorie,” “diet,” or “light” items on their menu. Even the cruise ships, those bastions of nonstop eating, now offer “healthy” choices on their menus.

If the main course portions are extremely generous or look rich and fattening, **order an appetizer instead of an entrée, or share an entrée with a friend.**

Day 286

Dessert

Desserts, as a rule, are rich in butter, cream, chocolate or sugar, and are concentrated sources of fat and calories.

Eating dessert is just a learned habit. Over time you can gradually change it to an occasional indulgence only.

Avoid the calorie-laden, fattening desserts. Order delicious arrays of cut-up fresh fruit or fresh berries so elegantly served in stemware.

Day 287

Dining Out

If the restaurant carries your favorite entrée in enormous servings, while placing your order, ask the waiter to put half of it in a special container, and take it home with you. Plan to have that portion for a meal the next day.

If you are dining with a friend who shares your health concerns and has made a similar commitment to sensible eating, inform the waiter ahead of time and **share the entrée or entire meal with your supportive friend.**

Day 288

Buying Food

As consumers, you are entitled to know the content of the foods on the supermarket shelves. Processed and prepared foods are required by law to list ingredients and nutritional information on the packaging.

Before purchasing or consuming prepared foods, **make a habit of reading the labels on packages of frozen, processed, or canned foods, to have a better idea of not only calories per serving but also total fat, saturated fat, cholesterol, and salt content.**

Day 289

Storing Food

Store all edibles out of sight and away from easy reach. Keep the snacks in the pantry, the kitchen cabinets, or the refrigerator.

Do not display the cookie jar, the cake plate, or the candy dish on the counter where they are visible and accessible at all times.

A basket or bowl of fresh fruit would be a welcome alternative, offering healthy choices.

Day 290

Serving Food

When you were a child, the adults who raised you were in a position of authority to decide the types of food you ate and the amounts you were served. They then demanded you "finish your food." As a result you developed the habit of eating everything on your plate, regardless of preferences, hunger, or need.

It is time to take charge. You select and choose the types of food you should eat, decide the amount you should have, and help yourself accordingly.

Day 291

On Vacation

Make sure you inform the other members in your party ahead of time that you intend to incorporate a brisk walk, tennis game, or other activity in your daily schedule. Plan to complete your workout early in the morning in order not to interfere with the group's plans for the day.

Stick with your plan.

Involve your friends where possible. Invite them to join you for your morning walk. You will have done them a great service by introducing them to a new healthier lifestyle.

Day 292

Reflections

Mastering the facts and accumulating the information is worthless unless it is put to good use. Most overweight people know exactly what to do to lose weight. Practice the new desirable habits until they become second nature to you.

Stop blaming others for your problem, stop finding excuses for being overweight, and stop depending on others for answers. **You will finally lose the weight only when you take full responsibility and take the reins.**

Day 293

Goal

The longest journey begins with one small step and is accomplished by a series of small steps all in the right direction.

Break down your target objective into short-term goals to make it easier for you to attain your goal. Divide this important project into simple and rewarding steps.

Determine the total number of pounds you intend to lose. Then, based on one or two pounds a week, chart a schedule for yourself to lose the weight slowly and steadily, just as you gained it.

Day 294

Rewards

Rewards work as strong positive incentives in reinforcing your new desirable habits, and they empower you to go on.

The most meaningful reward is the gratification felt upon accomplishment of a challenge, or the realization of a self-determined goal.

You must be very proud of yourself—the evolving, trim, and energetic person. Well done!

Day 295

Protein

Eating excessive amounts of protein does not "build" muscle, nor does it "firm up" muscle. The only way to increase body muscle mass and body strength is to exercise the muscles regularly.

Strength training or weight training helps build muscle, increases relative muscle mass in the body, elevates basal metabolic rate, burns up more calories, and slows down bone loss—osteoporosis.

Day 296

Fish

When buying canned tuna, salmon, or sardines, choose the water-packed variety, rather then the ones packed in oil. You will save around 200 fat calories per serving.

Enhance the taste with lots of fresh lemon juice, and add your favorite spices and condiments for a rich flavor.

For sandwiches, skip the mayonnaise, use generous amounts of lettuce, tomatoes, celery, cucumbers, and other favorite vegetables.

Mmm, good!

Day 297

Cheese

As a general rule, softer, creamier varieties of cheeses, such as Brie, Camembert, cream cheese, and ricotta, have a higher fat content compared to the hard cheeses. This fact should prompt you to select the hard cheeses over the soft varieties when offered a choice.

Instead of serving cheese in large chunks, use it as a condiment to increase the protein content, and to enhance the flavor of pastas, casseroles, salads, and sandwiches.

Day 298

Food Preparation Methods

One cannot overemphasize the fact that the way food is prepared is crucial in preserving the nutritional value of the natural and healthy raw materials, and determining as to whether a particular meal is healthy and low in calories or laden with fat and calories.

At a fast-food restaurant, fish fillet or chicken nuggets might sound healthier than a cheeseburger, but because they are batter fried, often in animal fat, you will end up getting twice as much fat and calories. Order the grilled chicken sandwich or one of the salads.

Day 299

Compare—and Make the Right Choices

Starbucks drinks, grande, 16 oz	Calories
Water, seltzer, club soda	0
Diet soda	4
Coffee, black	0
Coffee, one liquid creamer	60
Cappuccino with skim milk	110
Caramel Macchiato with skim milk	190
Caffe Mocha with skim milk	240
Cappuccino with whole milk	180
Caramel Macchiato with whole milk	250
Caffe Mocha with whole milk	420

Stick with skim milk, skip the whipped cream and syrup, order the smaller servings.

Day 300

Prevention

It is easier, healthier, and more desirable to **prevent obesity** than to deal with it after it develops. You are doing a lifelong favor to your family members, especially your children, by establishing the right eating habits and food preferences early on in life. You are the positive role model leading them to a healthier lifestyle, with lower risks of high blood pressure, heart disease, diabetes, some forms of cancer, and a host of other medical problems.

They will be grateful to you for life. You have earned a well-deserved pat on the back.

Day 301

Fiber

Bran is a good source of fiber and helps reduce blood cholesterol levels. Add it to your cereal or eat cereals enriched with bran.

The bran muffins available at bakeries or on pastry shelves claiming "high fiber" or "no cholesterol" are not necessarily beneficial or wholesome. Some contain more fat, sugar, and calories than rich desserts, and hence the beneficial effects of bran are offset by the added fat and calories.

Prepare your own muffins with skim milk, egg whites, and a fraction of the sugar, oil, or butter indicated in the recipe.

Day 302

Suggested Substitutions

Instead of	Use
Meat—pork, beef	Chicken, fish, beans
Milk—whole, low-fat	Skim milk
Peanuts, cashews	Cut-up fresh vegetables
Potatoes—mashed	Baked potatoes
Potato chips	Air-popped popcorn
Sour cream	Yogurt
Tuna, packed in oil	Tuna, packed in water
Yogurt—whole milk	Low-fat yogurt
Yogurt with jelly and jam	Yogurt with fresh fruit

Day 303

Salt

There is too much salt in processed, canned, or frozen prepared foods, and especially snacks.

Do your own cooking and baking, using reduced amounts of salt, and rely heavily on fresh vegetables and fruit.

Many canned vegetables, soups, broths, frozen prepared foods, and baked goods are now available in low-salt versions also. Select the reduced salt versions over the regular ones.

Day 304

Calories

Diets that prescribe a restricted menu, and list the specific food items that you are supposed to eat, do not allow any flexibility, and force you to eat foods you neither like nor want. You desperately wait for the day when this painful "sacrifice" will end.

But when you get "off the diet," you will revert right back to your old eating habits and the pounds will invariable creep back.

Design your own menu. Prepare your favorite meals with reduced fat, less animal protein, more vegetables, and savor the healthy meals you really enjoy.

Day 305

Physical Activity

Exercise is an effective factor in the reduction of the risk of osteoporosis, which is characterized by decreased bone mass and increased susceptibility to bone fractures, especially in older women.

Regular exercise, along with sufficient calcium from skim milk, fat-free yogurt, low-fat cottage cheese or supplements, helps in the prevention of osteoporosis.

If you are slacking off, visualize success. Close your eyes and see yourself as the trim, active, healthy and energetic person that you desire to be. Then go work out!

Day 306

Hunger

Hunger is a feeling that we all want to avoid or alleviate immediately, no matter how determined we are to lose the extra weight.

The feeling of fullness plays a major role in our food satisfaction, because once the stomach is full, our need for food diminishes.

Bulk alone is known to alleviate hunger. Eating foods based on the Superpyramid will satisfy hunger with optimal nutrition, minimal fat, and abundant fiber.

Three cheers for legumes, vegetables, and fruit!

Day 307

Healthy Eating Pyramid

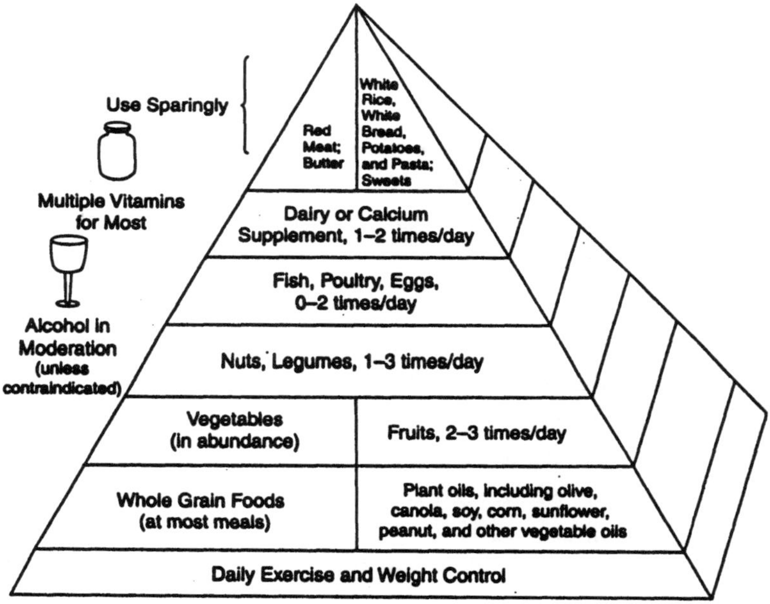

(From Willett, Walter C., MD, *Eat, Drink and Be Healthy,* Simon & Schuster, New York, 2001. Reprinted with permission.)

Day 308

Advantages of the *Healthy Eating Pyramid*

Incorporates physical activity and places daily exercise and weight control on the first level, the foundation of the pyramid, as the top priority. The lower and more stable your weight, the lower your chances of having high blood pressure, heart attacks, other types of cardiovascular disease, stroke, or diabetes.

Distinguishes between refined-grain carbohydrates and whole-grain carbohydrates. Whole-grain foods constitute the foundation of the diet. Brown rice, whole-wheat pasta, whole-grain bread, beans and other legumes are placed on the second tier, to be eaten at most meals. Highly refined or simple carbohydrates, such as white rice, white bread, pasta, and all sweets are placed at the top among the foods to be "used sparingly."

Day 309

Advantages of the *Healthy Eating Pyramid,* Continued

Differentiates between saturated fats and unsaturated fats: Fats from nuts, seeds, grains, fish, and liquid oils, including olive, canola, soybean corn, sunflower and peanut, are good and should be included in a wholesome diet. Saturated fats such as red meat, whole-milk dairy products, butter, and hydrogenated vegetable oils are banished to the top in the "use sparingly" category.

Separates protein sources into different categories: Proteins that come from plant sources are the healthiest. Nuts, beans, and other legumes are placed on the fourth level, to form the mainstay of food for protein. Fish, poultry, and eggs, the healthier of the animal proteins, are placed on the fifth level. Red meat is placed at the top in the "use sparingly" section because of its high saturated fat content.

Recommends taking a multivitamin daily.

Day 310

Dinner Parties

Stay away from all the fried hors d'oeuvres, dripping with oil and fat, that are being passed around. Those appetizers—such as batterfried mozzarella cheese fingers—are terribly rich in calories and could easily add up to more than your main course.

If you see a favorite item, by all means go ahead, help yourself and enjoy it, but eat a smaller portion of the main course and dessert.

Stay in control at all times; do not get carried away.

Day 311

On Vacation

Almost all hotels have swimming pools and fitness rooms fully equipped with the latest in exercise equipment. Put them to good use. Even on cruises there are reserved walking decks, pools, and exercise rooms.

Take in the museums and sightseeing attractions that require walking.

Join a "nature hike" group for a walk on special trails through the park.

Rent a bicycle and tour the area.

Go swimming or beach-combing instead of sunbathing for hours.

Day 312

Vegetarian Superpyramid

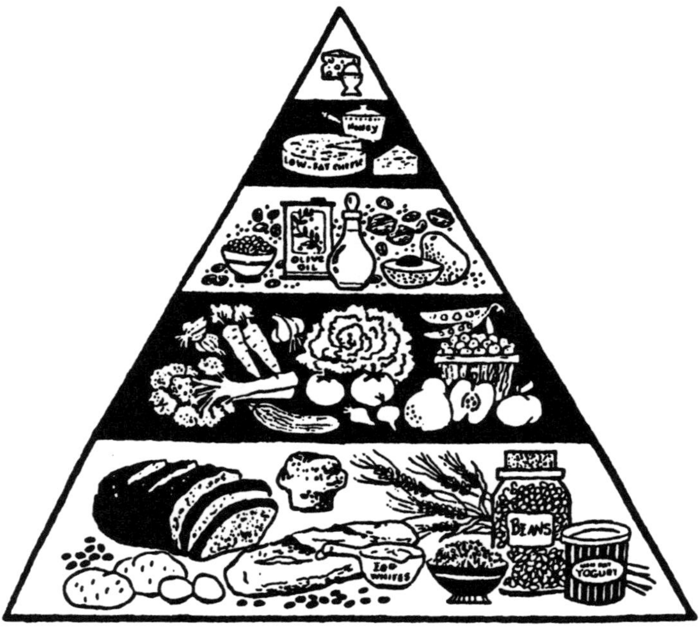

The main distinction is that eggs, cheese, yogurt, beans, and legumes constitute the source of protein.

(From Spiller, Gene, Ph.D., *The SuperPyramid Eating Program.* New York: Random House, 1993. Reprinted by permission of the Sphera Foundation and Gene Spiller.)

Day 313

Storing Food

Store fattening food and desserts in covered opaque containers and place them behind the low-calorie items in the refrigerator.

Keep low-calorie items in the most visible and accessible first rows in the pantry and kitchen cabinets.

For a healthy snack, peel carrots, cut into four sticks lengthwise, place in a clear container, cover with water, and keep in the refrigerator at eye level, front row.

Day 314

"Finish Your Food"

Think back on family dinner scenes when "cleaning your plate" was a big issue. How did you feel during those incidents? Do you still force yourself to finish it all?

Learn to trust your own judgment. Stop eating as soon as you decide that you have had enough, not when your plate is cleaned.

Feel comfortable about leaving some food on your plate, without feeling guilty about the children starving somewhere in the world. You should never be forced to eat one unnecessary excessive bite.

Day 315

Reinforcement

Choose your friends carefully. It is essential that you socialize with people who do not focus on food or make eating their primary preoccupation.

Spend time with individuals who care about their health, are selective in their eating habits, and are activity enthusiasts.

Cultivate friendships with people with whom you share a love of music, sports, books, crafts, hiking, and hobbies other than gourmet cooking and wine-tasting.

Day 316

Protein

Excess protein consumed is not stored by the body in the form of protein in larger muscles, but is metabolized and broken down to be used for energy. Any protein in excess of the energy requirements of the body is metabolized and stored as fat.

Excessive amounts of protein do not make adults any "stronger," or "more muscular."

Day 317

Eggs

Eggs are an excellent source of protein for children and young women in general, as well as for adults with no cholesterol-related health problems. The high-cholesterol content of egg yolks is well documented. Therefore adult men, older women, and individuals with high blood cholesterol levels should eat eggs sparingly.

For an occasional treat, you can prepare an omelet using one egg and the whites of two additional eggs, and a variety of chopped vegetables.

Day 318

Sugar

No artificial sweetener has been shown to help people lose weight or keep it off. Moreover, saccharine was shown to have life-threatening side effects, and the long-term effects of Aspartame (Nutra-Sweet and Equal) are not yet known.

Gradually reduce the amount of "diet" sodas that you drink; replace them with water, carbonated water, spring water, unsweetened fresh fruit juices, and unsweetened iced tea, flavored with fresh lemon juice.

Day 319

Behavior

If you suddenly get a strong craving for a rich snack that would ruin your daily calorie "budget plan," **decide to wait a half hour. In the meantime, keep busy.**

If at work, concentrate at the responsibility at hand. If at home, do your chores, make a phone call, read, write a letter, immerse yourself in one of your favorite hobbies, exercise, or go for a walk.

Getting your mind off the snack and physically away from it will help pass the urge. You will regain the upper hand, be in control, and might not want it after all.

Day 320

Fiber

Instead of drinking a glass of:	Eat
Orange juice 110 cal.	an orange 70 cal.
Grapefruit juice 95 cal.	a grapefruit 80 cal.
Apple juice 115 cal.	an apple 90 cal.

You will have the added pleasure of chewing, texture, longer taste, the satisfaction of more bulk, and the additional bonus of healthy fiber.

Day 321

Calories

Make sure your daily calorie intake does not go below 1200, for women and people of small stature, or 1500 for men and persons of large and tall bone structure.

If you go on an extremely low-calorie diet for a considerable time, your body responds to the apparent "starvation" and, in an effort to conserve energy, compensates by lowering the metabolic rate. Your metabolism slows down and fewer calories are used up to perform the same functions.

Day 322

Calories

If the perceived “starvation” continues over a period of weeks, the calorie-conservation mechanism can be so effective that weight loss will virtually stop. Worse yet, when you get off the crash diet, because your body is burning off fewer calories than before, you will end up with a larger excess of calories, will store more fat than before, and will gain the weight back faster.

Do not go on “starvation” diets, but persist with your new habit of eating reduced portions.

Day 323

Jogging

Jogging is a more strenuous version of walking. It has all the conveniences and benefits of walking and burns even more calories. Twenty to thirty minutes of jogging brings about the same benefits as forty to fifty minutes of fast walking. But jogging can be hard on the joints, especially in overweight people, and can lead to pain and injuries.

For an effective outdoor workout, you can alternate walking and jogging by walking uphill and jogging downhill. Give it a try!

Day 324

Physical Activity

Regular physical activity helps in the prevention and treatment of cardiovascular problems. It will heal and strengthen the heart by increasing blood circulation in the heart muscle and will reduce high blood pressure by improving overall blood circulation throughout the body.

Exercise reduces the incidence of heart disease and enhances general fitness and health.

Day 325

Salt

Use minimal amounts of salt in the food that you cook for your family members, so they do not develop a taste for excessive salt.

The taste of the foods children are raised with determines what they consider "delicious" as adults. These low-salt dishes will be their favorite meals, rich with the distinct flavors of the particular foods.

You will have given them the precious gift of healthier lives.

Day 326

Rate Your Weight

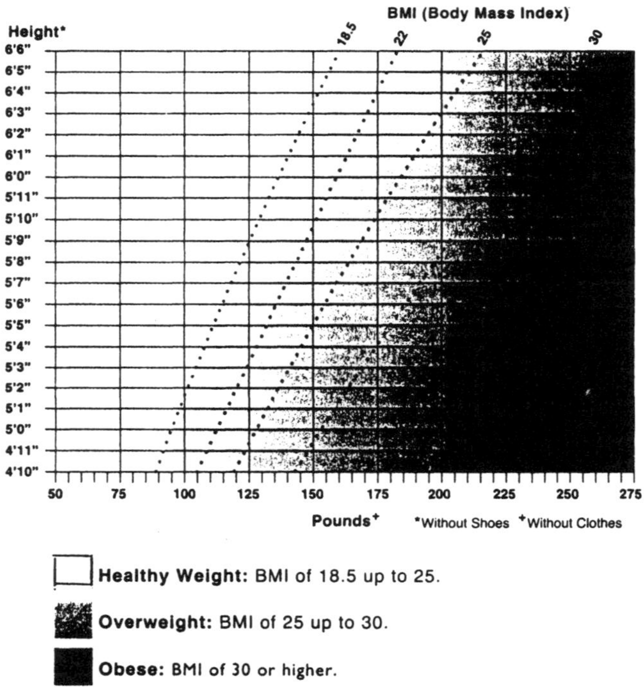

Body Mass Index (BMI)

Source: Dietary Guidelines for Americans, 2000. U.S. Department of Agriculture and U.S. Department of Health and Human Services. (Reprinted with permission.)

BMI gauges your weight in relation to your height. Which group do you fall into?

Day 327

Good Eating Habits

Use your diary as a guide for improvement. Review your weight control records regularly.

If a pattern emerges that points to a certain time of day, such as the afternoon or late evening, when you feel the strong urge for something to eat, plan for it ahead of time.

To avoid reaching for a calorie-laden food that happens to be available, set aside a healthy snack for that time slot and enjoy eating it slowly, relishing every morsel, without the slightest tinge of guilt.

Drink lots of water before and after eating.

Day 328

Good Eating Habits

If you have developed the habit of stopping at a certain bakery or candy store on your way to or from work, change your route.

If you routinely stop at a beckoning candy bar vending machine in one of the hallways on your way to or from your office, use another access route, avoid the temptation completely, and discontinue the habit for good.

Day 329

In Control

If you have a sudden urge to eat a serving of your favorite dessert in the middle of the day, delay the eating and promise yourself you will have some for dessert after dinner. When instead of thinking "I can't have that," you think "I will have it later on," you will not feel deprived, nor will you resent the thought of "forbidden foods."

Instead of feeling that you are making the utmost sacrifice, you will be in control and will feel good about yourself.

After dinner, enjoy every tiny bite of the anticipated dessert, if you still want it.

Day 330

Dinner Parties

Sit elegantly at a distance from the snacks for which you have a weakness. If the peanuts and potato chips are within your reach, you will be helping yourself the entire evening. But you will think twice before you get up from your chair and walk across the room to get a handful of nuts.

A mere four ounces of chips will add 650 calories, while four ounces of nuts will cost you 800 calories.

Day 331

Dinner Parties

Budget your total calories ahead of time.

Take all you decide to eat the first time around, remembering to reserve some calories for the fruit that you will have at dessert time.

No second helpings. Be assertive and firm. Learn to refuse food effectively and gracefully when pressured.

Day 332

Storing Leftovers

Put leftovers away immediately following the meal, while you are still full and satisfied.

Whenever possible, have someone else remove, store, or throw away leftovers so you won't have the temptation to nibble while putting them away.

Place single serving portions in individual containers, label, and store in the freezer.

Day 333

Rewards

You might have thought of yourself as a fat person for so long that you could have developed and accepted that image of yourself. Even though now you have lost a lot of weight, you might still perceive yourself as a fat person.

Now that the slimmer and activity-oriented person within you is emerging, adapt your mental image of yourself and proudly embrace the new trim and energetic winner you have become.

Day 334

Reinforcement

Celebrate your new improved image, show off your new trimmer figure, and visualize yourself as an even slimmer person in the future. This positive and joyous attitude keeps you from reverting to your old eating habits, and empowers you to continue forging forward.

This is the real you. The new trimmer, energetic, happier, confident, glamorous you.

You have worked wonders!

Day 335

Rewards

Now that your clothes feel loose on your slimmer figure, alter them to fit you better. Take them in at the seams, as tangible evidence of your achievement.

To stress your life-long commitment to your new lifestyle, and to assure your determination to attain your goal, and maintain it, cut out the extra material taken in.

Day 336

Stock Your Refrigerator with:

—Salad ingredients
—Fresh vegetables
—Whole-grain breads, English muffins
—Fat-free or low-fat salad dressing
—Fat-free or low-fat cottage cheese
—Fat-free or low-fat yogurt
—Some low-fat or fat-free cheese
—Spiced mustard, balsamic vinegar

Day 337

Stock Your Pantry with:

—Beans—all kinds (dry or canned)
—Chickpeas
—Lentils
—Split peas
—Brown rice
—Whole-wheat pasta
—Cracked wheat
—Canned tomatoes (crushed)
—Chicken broth (low-fat, fat-free cans)
—Extra virgin olive oil
—Onions
—Garlic
—Popcorn kernels

Day 338

Stock Your Freezer with Frozen:

—Corn kernels
—Peas
—Spinach—chopped
—Carrots—sliced
—String beans
—Mixed vegetables
—Sugar-free berries
—Sliced fruit
—Fat-free frozen yogurt (check sugar, calories)

Day 339

Weight Maintenance

You have arrived! You have achieved what you set out to do. Congratulate yourself. You have earned the right to boast. Go ahead, show off!

You have advanced to weight maintenance, which is achieved when the energy from food intake is equal to the sum total of energy expenditure by the essential body functions and the additional physical activity.

Body weight will remain stable when this balance is maintained.

Day 340

Maintenance

For most people, maintenance means keeping their weight at the desired reduced level with minimal fluctuation, by controlling calories.

Maintenance, however, is not limited just to calorie or energy balance. In order to successfully control weight, it also implies maintenance of the healthy lifestyle behavior, healthy eating patterns, good exercise habits, healthy attitude for life, and healthy interpersonal relationships.

Day 341

Weight Maintenance

Weight maintenance can be achieved by:

—Following consistently the eating behavior patterns learned and adopted on this program.
—Persisting in applying the nutritional information acquired.
—Continuing the regular physical activity. And
—Diligently keeping track of food and total calorie intake on a regular basis.

Day 342

Weight Maintenance

You have already developed a sense of desirable servings; you help yourself accordingly and find it quite satisfying.

You are now routinely choosing wholesome meals over the greasy alternatives, and you find it thoroughly enjoyable.

You are engaging in your favorite activity and find it most rewarding.

If on occasion you feel that you need some reinforcement, resort to keeping meticulous records for a while, until you get back on track.

Day 343

Weight Maintenance

You have now become a firm believer in the necessity of regular, consistent physical activity not only for weight reduction and maintenance, but also for the additional benefits of improved muscle tone, better overall fitness, increased energy, and enhanced general health.

Make sure that you continue the healthy pattern of regular physical activity.

Day 344

Weight Maintenance

Having experimented with various possible forms of exercise, you have by now determined the one physical activity that is the most convenient, practical, beneficial, and enjoyable for you.

Make that a pleasant experience; enjoy the activity and look forward to it as a natural and integral part of your daily routine for good.

Day 345

Weight Maintenance

Sports and games offer the wholesome activity in which family members of all ages can participate, enjoy, and benefit from the opportunity to improve their skills, learn from each other, and experience constructive competition.

Involve family members in your activity. You will be setting a great example for other adults to follow. The children will adopt the desirable practice early on and will develop life-long good habits.

Day 346

Weight Maintenance

Having young children should not keep you from your activities:

—Strap the baby to your chest or back when you go for your regular walk.
—Take the toddler along in a stroller, and stick to your regimen of power walking or jogging.
—Use a special bicycle seat and helmet for the child, and continue with your cycling.

Day 347

Weight Maintenance

Plan ahead for unusual situations, such as a business trip or a vacation, and be prepared to make the necessary adjustments to eliminate possible problems.

If you will be attending several luncheon meetings and dinner functions, plan ahead to choose the "light," low-fat, or vegetarian entrée, or order an appetizer instead of a full meal. Skip dessert entirely.

Increase your physical activity routine.

Day 348

Weight Maintenance

Make your own list of the most helpful ideas, information, habits or tips that you have found effective for your personal needs. Keep it handy.

Keep a copy of your "magic list" in your pocket appointment calendar. Post copies of you "most helpful tips" at visible spots in the kitchen so you can refer to it frequently for support and reinforcement.

Day 349

Weight Maintenance

There will be occasions when people who love you and mean well will offer you fattening foods and try to induce you to eat, thinking they are doing you a favor.

Stick to your long-term plans and habits. Let them know you appreciate their concern and thank them for their thoughtfulness, but refuse them politely and firmly.

You will feel wonderful. They will admire you for your determination and respect you more because of it.

Day 350

Weight Maintenance—Rewards

—You set out to achieve a goal and you did it. You are a winner.
—Be proud of yourself and your accomplishment.
—Admire the energetic, confident person that you see in the mirror every morning.
—Pat yourself on the back.
—Keep up the good work. You are doing great!

Day 351

Children

Congratulations!

Making healthy food choices, practicing good eating habits, and exercising regularly have become second nature to you now. The time has come for you to focus on setting a good example for your children and guiding them in developing these healthy habits.

Children naturally tend to follow parents in terms of exercise and eating habits. Be a positive role model and help them grow in an environment where healthy habits are practiced as the norm.

Habits formed in childhood will last a lifetime.

Day 352

Children

The percentage of obese children in the United States is dangerously high and is still increasing at an alarming rate.

Clinical studies show that the first evidence of coronary heart disease—fatty deposits in the coronary arteries—begins appearing at an early age in children eating the typical American diet. During the teenage years, the high-fat fast foods consumed only exacerbate the condition.

Many major health problems confronting adults today can be traced back to eating and activity habits established during childhood.

Day 353

Children

Studies show that heart disease is virtually absent in Asian or African rural cultures where the typical diet is low in fat content throughout life.

The majority of cases of coronary artery disease can be prevented by **significant reductions in dietary fat if implemented early in life.**

Day 354

Children

Adult children of immigrants from China and Japan who grew up in the United States and adopted the typical American high-fat diet, have the same high rate of heart disease as other American adults, in contrast to the adults still living in China and Japan.

The higher incidence of heart disease appears in the very first generation with the fat-laden high cholesterol diet consumed from early childhood.

Day 355

Children

Children are not born with a taste for animal fat. It is a learned habit.

Lifetime eating habits are established early on, and an eating pattern is set for the rest of an individual's life.

Adults who are afflicted with cardiovascular disease and some forms of cancer are suffering in part because of what they ate while growing up.

Day 356

Children

Clinical studies have shown that among adults, the high blood cholesterol levels and coronary artery deposits can be reduced with a drastic drop in the consumption of dietary fat, slowing down the progress of heart disease, or relieving symptoms.

Similarly, reducing children's dietary fat lowers their blood cholesterol levels within weeks, showing a significant drop in a few months.

Day 357

Children

Apply the knowledge you now possess to **prevent** diseases that your children will have to cure later on as adults.

Give them the great gift of good eating habits. Lead them early on to the path of healthy food preferences so these become second nature for them too.

It is a learned process that will affect their health and well-being for the rest of their lives.

Day 358

Children

Overweight children are more likely to become overweight adults, with increased risk of heart disease.

Excessive body fat accumulating during infancy, and later on during adolescence, not only enlarges the existing fat cells but also **increases the number of permanent fat cells. Weight loss in adults just reduces the size of the cells. The number of fat cells is not reduced. Thus obese children will have a greater tendency to become overweight adults.**

Day 359

Children

Children grow up imitating the dietary habits of the adult members of the family. These eating habits are passed on from one generation to the other, if no effort is made to improve the pattern.

There certainly is a definite genetic factor involved, but lifestyle habits of consuming excessive dietary fat and animal flesh, and exercising too little are major factors that lead to obesity, adult onset diabetes, high blood pressure, and heart disease.

You play a vital role in your children's future. Give them the gift of healthier lives from the start.

Day 360

Children

Toddlers share the meals of their family members and develop a taste for whatever satisfies their hunger; they learn to think of those items as “good” and “tasty” food.

Help them acquire a taste for foods low in fat, low in salt and sugar, rich with complex carbohydrates, and plentiful with vegetables. Let them learn that fruit is the best treat and the most delicious dessert.

Day 361

Children

Animal protein sources contain high levels of fat, saturated fat, and cholesterol. They should be used sparingly.

Protein from a rich variety of vegetable sources is quite adequate and even healthier, with very low fat content.

Legumes—peas, lentils, chickpeas, and all varieties of beans—are excellent sources of protein. In addition, they are richer in fiber and more filling.

Day 362

Children

Offer your children generous servings of complex carbohydrates, the delicious vegetables that nature provides in abundance. The choice is staggering: potatoes, sweet potatoes, sweet corn, carrots, rice, cracked wheat, cereal, green beans, squash, broccoli, and asparagus, to name just a few.

Use sliced fresh fruit for a reward. Let them think of fruit as the ultimate treat.

Day 363

Children

Serve a salad with each meal. Eat a large helping of the salad with gusto. Let the children see you enjoying it thoroughly. Familiarize them with the many salad greens, tomatoes, celery, cucumber, red and green peppers, and other healthy fillers.

Prepare their sandwiches with just two thin slices of the cold cuts, one thin slice of cheese, and stuff the sandwiches to overflowing with lettuce, tomatoes, and cucumbers.

Day 364

Children

Involve the children in regular physical activity, especially if they are not participating in school or community team sports.

Limit television watching and discourage your children from eating in front of the television set.

Plan evening and weekend walks with each child individually, and make it a pleasant, bonding experience. Help them associate good feelings with these walks so they will look forward to them with joy and anticipation.

Plan weekend projects to revolve around family activities such as hiking, cycling, or swimming.

Day 365

Children

If your children are old enough, hold a family meeting before you make any sudden changes. Discuss with them the advantages of the dietary improvements that you are planning to institute.

You will get their full cooperation if they participate in the decision-making process and feel that they had a say in it.

Make it an exciting challenge. Implement changes gradually. Try new recipes. Make it fun and enjoyable.

Weight Chart

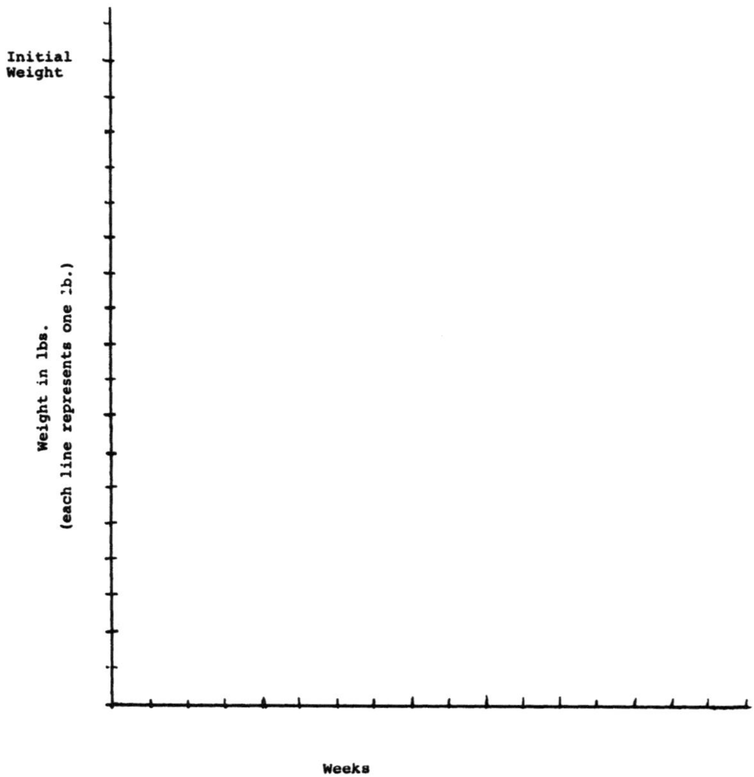

Calorie Guide to Some Basic Foods

Food	Approximate Calories
Almonds	
Whole, 1 cup	850
Roasted in oil, 1 cup	985
Roasted in oil, 1 ounce	180
Apple, raw, 1 medium	90
Apple cider, sweet, 8 oz	125
Apple juice, 1 cup	115
Applesauce	
Unsweetened, 1 cup	100
Sweetened, 1 cup	230
Asparagus, 1 cup	35
Avocado, California, 1 average, pitted	370
Diced, 1 cup	250
Mashed, 1 cup	390
Avocado, Florida, 1 average, pitted	200
Diced, 1 cup	190
Mashed, 1 cup	300
Bacon	
Cooked, 3 medium slices	130
Canadian, cooked, 2 slices	115
Bagel, 1 water	160
Banana, 1 medium	100
Beans	
Great northern, cooked, 1 cup	210
Kidney, cooked, 1 cup	220
Lima, cooked, 1 cup	190

Food	Approximate Calories
Green string, cooked, 1 cup	30
Yellow wax, cooked, 1 cup	30
Beef, 4 ounces	
Brisket, braised	470
Brisket, trimmed of fat, braised	250
Corned, boiled, medium fat	425
Ground, regular, broiled	325
Ground, lean, broiled	250
Porterhouse steak, broiled	530
Porterhouse, trimmed of fat, broiled	255
Rib roast, roasted	500
Rib roast, trimmed of fat, roasted	275
Roast	255
Sirloin steak, broiled	465
Sirloin steak, trimmed of fat, broiled	235
T-bone steak, broiled	540
T-bone steak trimmed of fat, broiled	255
Beets, cooked, 1 cup	70
Biscuits	
Medium, 1	130
Small, 1	85
Blackberries and blueberries	
Fresh, 1 cup	85
Canned, in syrup, 1 cup	230
Bouillon, beef or chicken, 2 cubes	10
Breads (check package label) 1 slice	45-90
Broccoli florets, 1 cup	50
Brussels sprouts, 1 cup	50
Butter, 2 tablespoons or 1 oz	220
Cabbage, green or red, 1 cup	30
Cakes	
Most cakes, no icing, 1 slice	160
Most cakes, iced, 1 slice	300
Chocolate devil's food, iced, 1 slice	440
Cupcakes, iced, one	170

Food	Approximate Calories
Candy (check label info.), 1 oz average	150
Cantaloupe, diced, 1 cup	65
Carrots, sliced, 1 cup	50
Cauliflower, 1 cup	30
Celery, diced 1 cup	20
Cereals (check box information)	
No sugar or milk added, 1 cup	140-200
1 cup, with ½ cup skim milk	180-340
Cheese (see Dairy)	
Chicken	
Broiled, no skin, 4 oz	190
Broiled, with skin, 4 oz	250
Fried, with skin, 4 oz	285
Roasted, no skin, 4 oz	210
Fried, 1 breast	160
Fried, 1 drumstick	90
Fried, 1 thigh	120
Fried, 1 wing	80
Chicken pot pie, small	545
Cocoa, all milk, 1 cup	175
Coffee, 1 cup	
Black	5
Black, with 2 tsp. sugar	35
With 1 tbsp. whole milk	15
With 1 tbsp. light cream	35
With 1 tsp. sugar and 2 tbsp. cream	65
Coleslaw, 1 cup	60
Corn	
Cooked, 1 ear	70
Cooked, 1 cup	135
Creamed, 1 cup	210
Cranberries, raw, 1 cup	45
Cranberry juice, 6 oz	125
Cranberry sauce, 1 cup	405
Cucumber, 1 medium	20
Custard, baked, 1 cup	305

Food	Approximate Calories
Dairy products	
Butter, 1 tbsp.	100
Butter, ½ cup, 1/4 lb 1 stick	815
Cheese, most, 1 oz (check package)	90-110
Cheese, cottage, 1% fat, 1 cup	160
Cheese, cottage, 2% fat, 1 cup	200
Cheese, cottage, 4% fat, 1 cup	280
Cream, half & half, 2 tbsp.	40
Cream, light, 2 tbsp.	65
Cream, light, ½ cup	255
Cream, light, whipping, ½ cup	360
Cream, heavy, ½ cup	420
Eggnog, all milk, 8 oz	290
Margarine, 1 tbsp.	100
Milk, fat-free, 1 cup	80
Milk, 1%, 1 cup	110
Milk, 2%, 1 cup	130
Milk, whole, 1 cup	160
Milk shake, chocolate, 8 oz	420
Milk shake, chocolate malted, 8 oz	500
Sour cream, 2 tbsp.	60
Sour cream, ½ cup	230
Yogurt, plain, from non-fat milk, 1 cup	110
Yogurt, plain, from whole milk, 1 cup	155
Yogurt, with fruit, 1 cup	260
Yogurt, vanilla flavored, 1 cup	200
Donuts	
Plain, 1	125
Sugared or iced, 1	150
Jelly, 1	225
Duck, roasted, 4 oz	370
Eclairs, custard filling, chocolate, 1	240
Egg, boiled whole, 1 large	80

Food	Approximate Calories
Fish, 4 oz servings	
Bass, broiled or baked, no fat	110
Bass, fried	220
Bluefish, broiled or baked with butter	180
Bluefish, fried	230
Cod fillet, broiled	190
Haddock, fried	190
Halibut, broiled with butter	190
Salmon, canned	160-230
Salmon, broiled, with butter	210
Salmon, smoked	200
Tuna, canned in water	145
Tuna, canned in oil, drained	225
Fruit cocktail, fruit salad	
Water packed, 1 cup	90
Syrup packed, 1 cup	195
Gelatin mold, fruit flavored, 1 cup	160
Gelatin mold, fruit added, 1 cup	300
Grapefruit (pink, red, or white)	
Fresh, 1 medium	80
Fresh, sections, 1 cup	95
Canned, sections, water pack, 1 cup	75
Canned, sections, syrup pack, 1 cup	180
Grapefruit juice, fresh, 1 cup	95
Grapes, most kinds, 1 cup	70-105
Grape juice, canned or bottled, 1 cup	135-165
Ham, 4 oz	
Light cure, lean roasted	215
Light cure, medium fat, roasted	330
Long cure, country-style, lean	355
Long cure, country-style	445
Hamburger, broiled, with bun, 2 oz	255
Hamburger, with 1 oz cheese and bun	365
Honey, 1 tbsp.	65

Food	Approximate Calories
Ice Cream, 1 cup	220-360
Ice Cream Soda, 8 oz	255
Ice milk, vanilla, 1 cup	180-240
Jams, jellies, fruit preserves, 1 tbsp.	55
Lamb, 4 oz	
Leg, roasted, trimmed of fat	210
Leg, roasted, fat not trimmed	320
Chops, trimmed of fat	225
Chops, fat not trimmed	400
Lentils, whole, cooked, 1 cup	210
Lettuce, most kinds, chopped, 1 cup	15
Liquor—Alcoholic Beverages	
Beer, light 12 oz	105
Beer, regular, 12 oz	155
Distilled spirits, 80 proof, 1 oz	70
Distilled spirits, 100 proof, 1 oz	85
Liqueurs and cordials, 1 oz	80-120
Mixed drinks, 4 oz	160-190
Wines, most kinds, 4 oz	80-130
Lobster, cooked, 1 cup	140
Lobster Newburg, 1 cup	485
Lox, 4 oz	200
Macaroni, cooked, 1 cup	155
Macaroni and cheese, baked, 1 cup	430
Margarine, 1 tbsp.	100
Margarine, 1 stick, 4 oz	815
Mayonnaise, 1 tbsp.	110
Melon, most kinds, cubed, 1 cup	50
Milk (see dairy products)	
Muffins (check package), most, 1	105-125
Mushrooms, sliced, 1 cup	20

Food	Approximate Calories
Nectarine, fresh, 1 medium	90
Noodles, egg, cooked, 1 cup	200
Nuts, a dozen mixed nuts	100
Cashews, roasted in oil, 1 cup	780
Macadamia, 6 nuts	105
Peanuts, roasted, shelled, 1 cup	840
Pecans, shelled, 1 cup	740
Pistachio, shelled, 1 cup	890
Walnuts, shelled, 1 oz	180
Walnuts, shelled, 1 cup	785
Oils, most vegetable oils, 1 tbsp.	100-120
Oranges, 1 medium	70
Orange juice, fresh, 1 cup	115
Pancake, small, 1	60
Pancake, large, 1	155
Peaches, fresh, whole, 1 medium	50
Canned, water pack, 1 cup	75
Canned, syrup pack, 1 cup	200
Peanut butter, 1 tbsp.	95
Pears, fresh, 1 medium	90
Canned, water pack, 1 cup	80
Canned, syrup pack, 1 cup	195
Peppers, green & red, fresh, sliced, 1 cup	25
Pies, most, 1 average serving	300-400
Pizza, baked, cheese, 1 large slice	130-200
Popcorn, air popped, plain, 1 cup	25
Popped in oil, 1 cup	40
Popped in oil, 1 tbsp. butter added, 1 cup	145
Pork, 4 oz	
Most cuts, cooked, trimmed of fat	290
Most cuts, cooked, with fat	430
Spareribs, fat not trimmed, braised	500

Food	Approximate Calories
Potatoes	
Baked or boiled, 1 medium	110
French fried, 10 strips	200
Fried, 1 cup	455
Hash brown, 1 cup	355
Scalloped, without cheese, 1 cup	255
Scalloped, with cheese, 1 cup	355
Potato chips, 10 chips	115
Potato chips, 2 oz	320
Potato salad, with mayonnaise, 1 cup	365
Prunes, dehydrated, uncooked, 1 cup	345
Puddings, most, 1 cup	320
Radishes, fresh, 10 medium	10
Raisins, packaged, 1 tbsp.	25
Raisins, packaged, 1 cup	420
Raspberries, red, fresh, 1 cup	70
Red, frozen sweetened, 1 cup	245
Black, fresh, 1 cup	100
Rice, 1 cup	
Brown, long grain, cooked	230
White, long grain, cooked	225
White, long grain, instant, cooked	180
Rice pudding, with raisins, 1 cup	386
Rolls and buns, most, 1	100
Danish pastry, plain, 1	310
Hoagie or submarine roll, 1 large	380
Salad dressings	
Most dietary brands, 2 tbsp.	20-40
Most regular brands, 2 tbsp.	130-160
Sandwich, 1, on white bread, plain	
Bacon (4 slices), lettuce, tomato	300
Bologna (2 oz) and cheese (1 oz)	355
Cheese, American or Cheddar (2 oz)	315
Chicken, roasted, 2 oz	195

Food	Approximate Calories
Chicken salad, 2 oz	245
Club (bacon, chicken, tomato, lettuce)	590
Egg, hard boiled, (½) and tomato (½)	150
Peanut butter, (2 tbsp.)	290
Peanut butter, (2 tbsp.), jelly (2 tbsp.)	345
Roast beef, (2 oz)	240
Salami, (2 oz), cheese (1 oz)	380
Tuna salad (2 oz)	280
Turkey, roasted (2 oz)	200
Sardines, oil pack, drained, 4 oz	230
Sausages and cold cuts, 1 oz	80-130
Shrimp, raw, shelled, 4 oz	100
Shelled, breaded, fried, 4 oz	255
Soft drinks	
Diet sodas, 12 oz	0-40
Regular sodas, 12 oz	100-150
Soups (consult can info.), 1 cup	
Chicken consommé	20
Bean	200
Clam chowder, Manhattan	75
Clam chowder, New England	175
Green pea, split pea	140
Mushroom, cream	135
Onion, French	125
Spaghetti, cooked, 1 cup	155-190
Spaghetti, cheese, tomato sauce, 1 cup	260
Spaghetti, meatballs, cheese, sauce, 1 cup	330
Spinach, fresh, chopped, 1 cup	15
Cooked, chopped 1 cup	40
Squash, baked, mashed, 1 cup	100-140
Strawberries, fresh, unsweetened, 1 cup	55
Frozen, sweetened, 1 cup	235
Sugar, granulated, 1 tsp.	15
Granulated, 1 tbsp.	45
Granulated, 1 cup	770

Food	Approximate Calories
Brown, loose, 1 cup	540
Brown, packed, 1 cup	820
Sweet potatoes, baked, boiled, 4 oz	125
Boiled in skin, mashed, 1 cup	290
Tangerine, 1 medium fruit	40
Tomato, fresh, 1 medium	25
Turkey, roasted, 4 oz	215
Roasted, chopped, 1 cup	265
Veal, 4 oz	
Loin, braised	265
Rib roast, braised	305
Breast, braised	345
Waffles, baked, plain, 1	90-130
Watermelon, diced, 1 cup	40
Zucchini, fresh, sliced, 1 cup	20
Boiled, mashed 1 cup	30